A *BOUQUET* OF
AROMA~
THERAPY

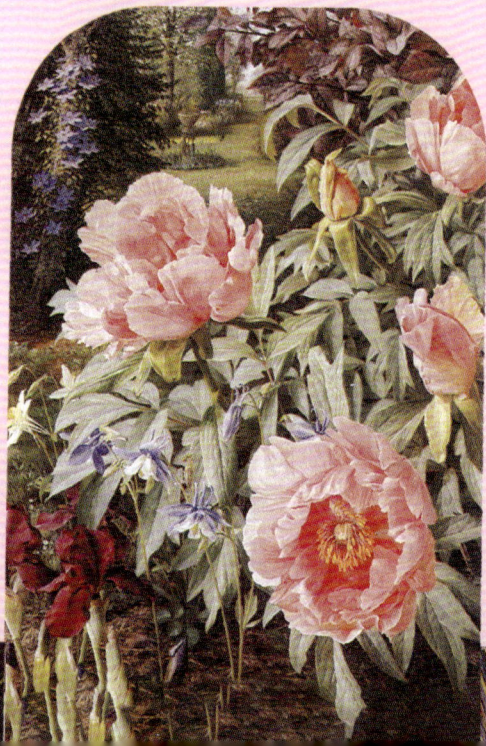

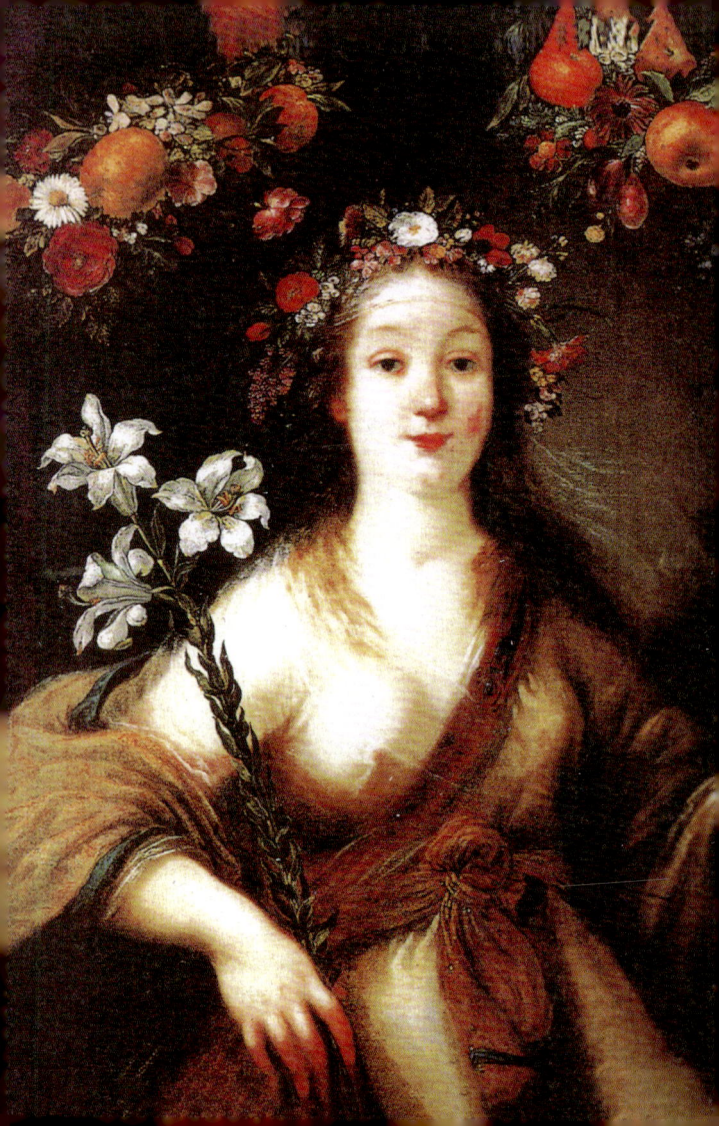

A GIFT OF HEALTH

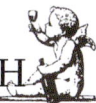

A *BOUQUET* OF

AROMA~ THERAPY

ESSENTIAL OILS & FRAGRANT MASSAGE, FLORAL REMEDIES & ELEGANT EXTRACTS

COMPILED AND
VISUALLY EMBELLISHED
FROM ORIGINAL SOURCES BY
W. CRAIG DODD ESQ.

IMM
lifestyle
books™

Read. Learn. Do What You Love.

Text, illustrations, and photographs by IMM Lifestyle Books, an imprint of Fox Chapel Publishing, 903 Square Street, Mount Joy, PA 17552. *www.foxchapelpublishing.com*

First published in 1996 by New Holland (Publishers) Ltd.

Designed and edited by
Complete Editions
40 Castelnau, London SW13 9RU

Editor: Michèle Brown
Designer: Craig Dodd
Editorial Direction: Yvonne McFarlane

ISBN 978-1-5048-0153-9

Printed in China
First Printing

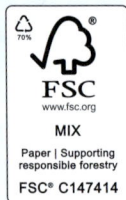

FSC
www.fsc.org

MIX

Paper | Supporting
responsible forestry

FSC® C147414

To learn more about the other great books from Fox Chapel Publishing, or to find a retailer near you, call toll-free at 800-457-9112 or visit us at *www.FoxChapelPublishing.com*. We are always looking for talented authors. To submit an idea, please send a brief inquiry to acquisitions@foxchapelpublishing.com.

Or write to:
Fox Chapel Publishing
903 Square Street
Mount Joy, PA 17552

This is not a medical book. It is a gift book. It is not intended to replace the services of a physician, nor is it meant to encourage diagnosis and treatment of illness, disease or other medical problems by the layman. Any application of the recommendations set out in the following pages is at the reader's discretion and sole risk. If under a physician's care, they will advise if any recommendations are suitable for you. Pregnant Women are advised to avoid all drugs—synthetic or herbal.

CONTENTS

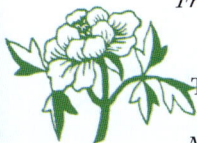

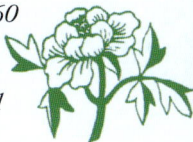

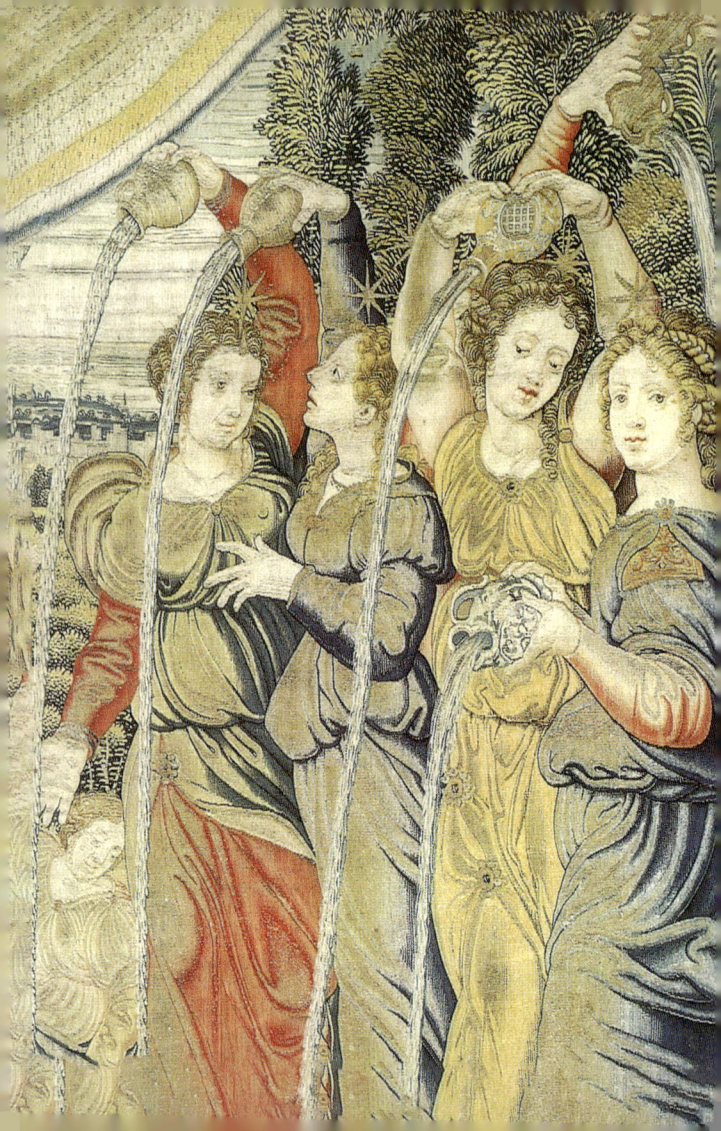

PREFACE

Within the pages of the Small Volumes which comprise of **A Gift of Health** there is contained the Collected Wisdom of Sages and Savants, Herbalists and Sensualists from throughout the Ages.

From their very Words the Modern Reader may glean much **Useful Information** to help with the **Problems of Everyday Life**, be they Physical or Psychological.

This very volume offers a Tantalizing Insight into a Particular World of **Life-Enhancing Wisdom**, as do the Companion Volumes.

A Garden of Herbal Remedies takes you along the Pathways of the Healing Herbal Garden. The Wisdom of the Ancient Herbalists being distilled to illuminate this Healing Art. The Potency of Each and Every Herb herein is defined, together with a Veritable Pharmacopoeia of Nature's Remedies to lead to a Healthier Life.

A Compendium of Oriental Healing takes you into the Erudite World of the Ancient Healing Arts of the Orient. The Mysteries of Acupuncture, Meditation, Moxibustion and the Oldest of Herbal Cures are explained, together with the Ways of Ayurvedic Medicine which treats the Whole Person rather than an Isolated Disease.

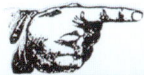

A Bouquet of Aromatherapy is a Celebration of the Healing, Soothing and Sensual Qualities of the Plant Kingdom. It offers a Perfumed Voyage through the World of Essential Oils, their Uses, Practical applications and Healing Properties. It also features Dr. Bach's famed Flower Remedies and, on a lighter note, the Creation of Personal Pot-pourri and Fragrances.

A Cornucopia of Aphrodisiacs combines many of the Features of the aforesaid Companion Volumes, bringing together Folklore and Fancy, Enchanting Elixirs and Arousing Recipes to Enhance the Libido and Promote a Joyful Union of Partners.

Taken together, ingested and digested, the Messages from Across the Aeons of Time will truly prove to be **A Gift of Health.**

W. Craig Dodd

The Author thanks Michael Mitchell Johnstone of that Ilk for his Painstaking Research without which this Estimable Volume would have remained Unwritten.

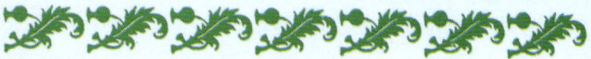

Floreat Therapia Aromaticum

What would a Rose Garden be without the Heady Bouquet of Opulent Blooms pregnant with perfume? An Orchard without the Scent of Apple Blossoms? A Beach without a Tang of Salt? A Mountainside without the Aroma of Heather? A Secret Romance without the Tantalizing Fragrance worn by the Object of One's Desires?

Smell is the Underused, but most Evocative of the Quintet of Senses that enrich our lives so. The slightest suspicion of an Evocative Scent can whisk us back to a long-ago holiday by the seaside when the world was young and every rock pool promised adventure. A hint of Particular Perfume quickens our heart's beat as we recall the joy of being in love for the first time, while the trace of another clouds the eyes with tears by bringing to mind parting from a loved one.

The most august of Lexicographies, the **Oxford English Dictionary**, defines aroma as the distinctive fragrance of a spice or plant, and therapy as curative treatment. Effect an introduction between these two, give them time to flirt a little and their betrothal when consummated is a range of fragrant remedies to revive our flagging spirits, soften our skins, add lustre to our hair and sparkle to our eyes, whilst generally enhancing our Lives in Total.

It is Little Wonder, as the world spins frantically into the uncertainty of a NewMillenium, that the fruit of the marriage of aroma and therapy has matured into one of the most popular of the healing arts – and surely the most creative.

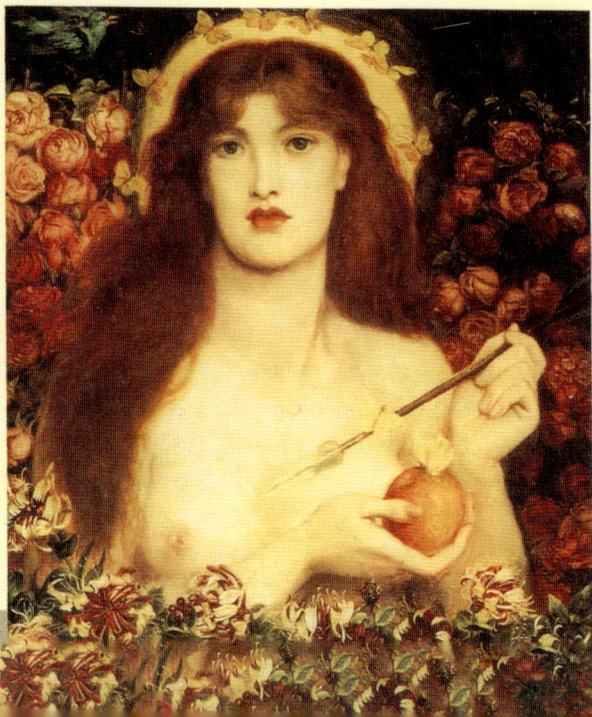

WHAT'S IN A WORD

In **Ancient Egypt,** as *Ra the Sun God* glowed red in the **Evening Sky**, priests burned a heady mixture of saffron, cassia, spikenard, cinnamon, juniper and eleven other wondrous ingredients to ensure his safe return in the **Eastern Skies** the following day.

The **Greeks** believed that their gods descended from Mount Olympus on **Perfumed Clouds** wearing robes redolent of fragrant essences. And it was there that the worthy and wise Hippocrats advocated the healthful benefits to be gained by adding scented oils to warm bath water. And remaining in the Groves of Arcady, Theophrastus wisely observed that 'Oils applied externally affect the body internally'.

The **Romans,** heirs to the Glory that was Greece, were profligate in their use of scented oils, none more so than **Dissolute Nero** who adorned himself with a twelve-month's supply of perfume when he watched his wife being carried to her final place of rest.

In the mysterious East, wealthy **Chinese** women were brought to confinement in a special room in which was burned the wood of the artemesia tree, the wafting fumes of which attracted kindred spirits and induced joy into mother and new-born child.

The Discovery of **Distillation** by the **Turks**, at the end of the tenth century and beginning of the eleventh, made easier the extraction of essential oils and yielded fluids of great purity which were later brought to Europe by Li-on-hearted Crusaders returning from the Holy Land.

Essential oils were widely used by such **Herbalists** as the esteemed **Culpeper** and **Gerard.** And despite the increasing **Knowledge** of **Chemistry** which resulted in herbals being cast in a Jaundiced Light, many continued to believe in the **Mystic Power** of **Perfume.** Marcel Proust journeyed from Paris to Normandy to Seek Inspiration by inhaling the scent of apple blossoms, while Schiller, his fellow worshipper at the temples of Calliope and her Sister Muse, Clio, inhaled the pungent aroma of rotting apples when he needed to find the Precise Word he was seeking.

Despite its Long and Distinguished History, **Aromatherapy** remained an unspoken word until the fourth decade of our present century when a French scientist, seeking relief from a burn, plunged his painful hand into a jar brimful with pure lavender oil. The speed with which his hand healed led him to research the properties of the essential oils and to coin the word, **Aromatherapy.**

Two other pioneers hailed from France – Jean Valnet and Marguerite Maury. M. Valnet treated wounded soldiers with essential oils and went on to become one of the Brightest Stars in Aromatherapy's Firmament. Mme Maury pioneered the use of diluted essential oils in body massage.

Aromatherapy technique has at last moved out of the receipt books and manuals of a Few Devotees into the mainstream of Modern Life.

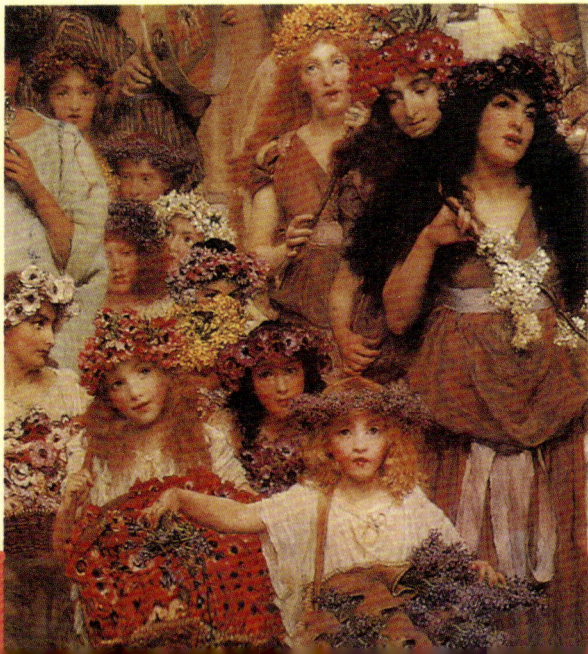

BASIL

Legend has it that Basil was found growing on the site of the Crucifixion by the Empress Helena who brought it back from Jerusalem to Greece. Since then the plant has flourished over many Mediterranean lands. In India, it is held in the highest regard, and is dedicated to Krishna and Vishnu, the second of the Hindu Trimurti.

Basil's distinctive, all-pervasive aroma is a clue that the oil it yields is one of the most powerful in the Aromatherapist's Armoury, an appropriate tribute for a plant whose name comes from the Greek *basileus*, meaning king. Such is the strength of oil this regal herb yields, it should only be used in the lowest concentrations.

Those whose Nerves are in need of a Tonic or who wish to stimulate their Thinking Powers will find Basil beneficial. It is a boon to anyone battling with Bronchitis and a help to those with troublesome Sinuses.

Basil's clove-like, liquorice aroma is an ideal complement to the Citrus oils, Frankincense, Geranium and Neroli, with all of which it blends beautifully.

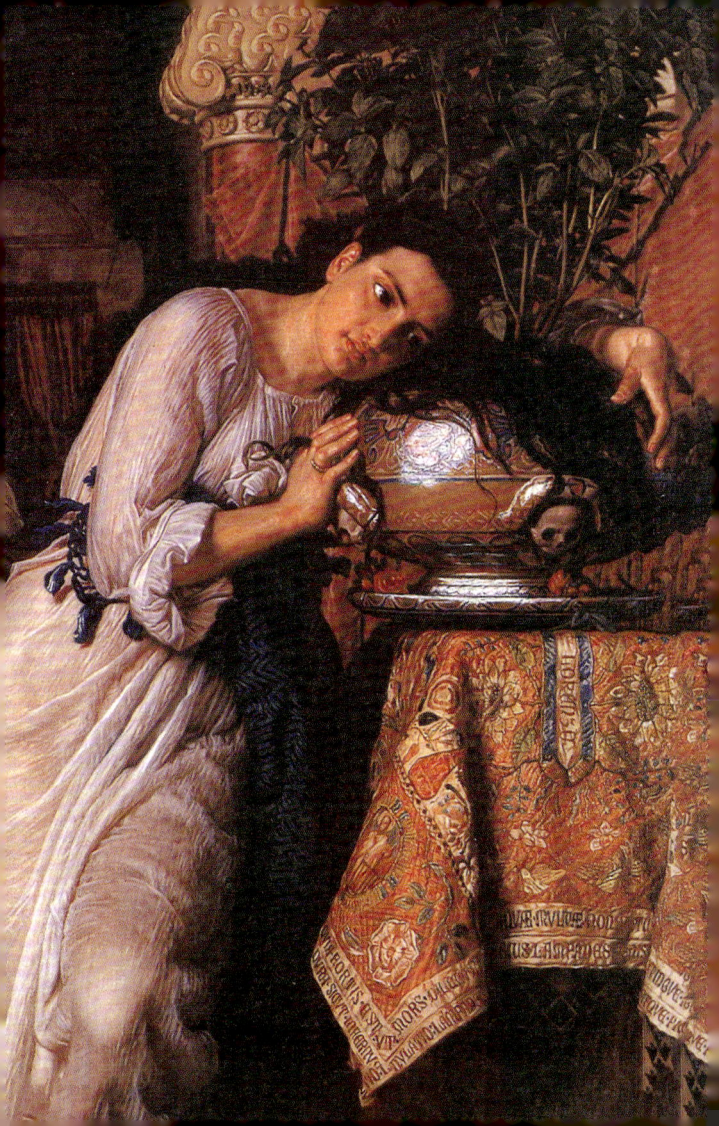

BERGAMOT

There are many who opine that the Bergamot tree takes its name from Bergamo, the town a few miles north of Milan where it was first cultivated. Those who disagree hold that it is from the Bey's pear, *beg-armundi*, once grown in Turkey, that the name has its genesis.

The tree, among the smallest in the **Citrus** arbour, is now mainly grown in Calabria and Sicily, and to a lesser extent, in the coastal groves of Morocco and Africa's Ivory Coast.

This deep emerald-green oil which is at once sweet, citric and floral, is among the most refreshing of all essential oils. It counters depression and uplifts the spirit. It is, too, a trusty antiseptic and dependable disinfectant.

Those seeking a suitable treatment for boils, spots and body ulcers, chicken pox, herpes and psoriasis will find that a few drops added to bathwater or onto a compress extremely efficacious. As an inhalant it lifts depression and relieves anxiety. But perhaps its most famous use is as a flavourant in the tea favoured by that most English of tea lovers, Earl Grey.

Caveat all who worship at the Temple of Helios

Because it increases the skin's sensitivity, Bergamot is commonly listed as being among the ingredients of many of the preparations applied by those who wish to darken their skin by exposure to sunlight. Ladies fortunate in being blessed with fair skin should shy from their use as there is a risk that such lotions encourage Pigmental Abnormalities. It is similarly unwise, indeed foolhardy, for even the swarthiest of men to apply Bergamot directly to the skin.

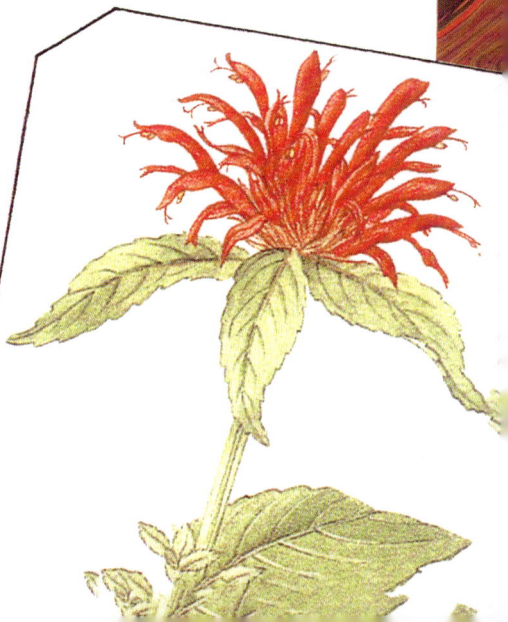

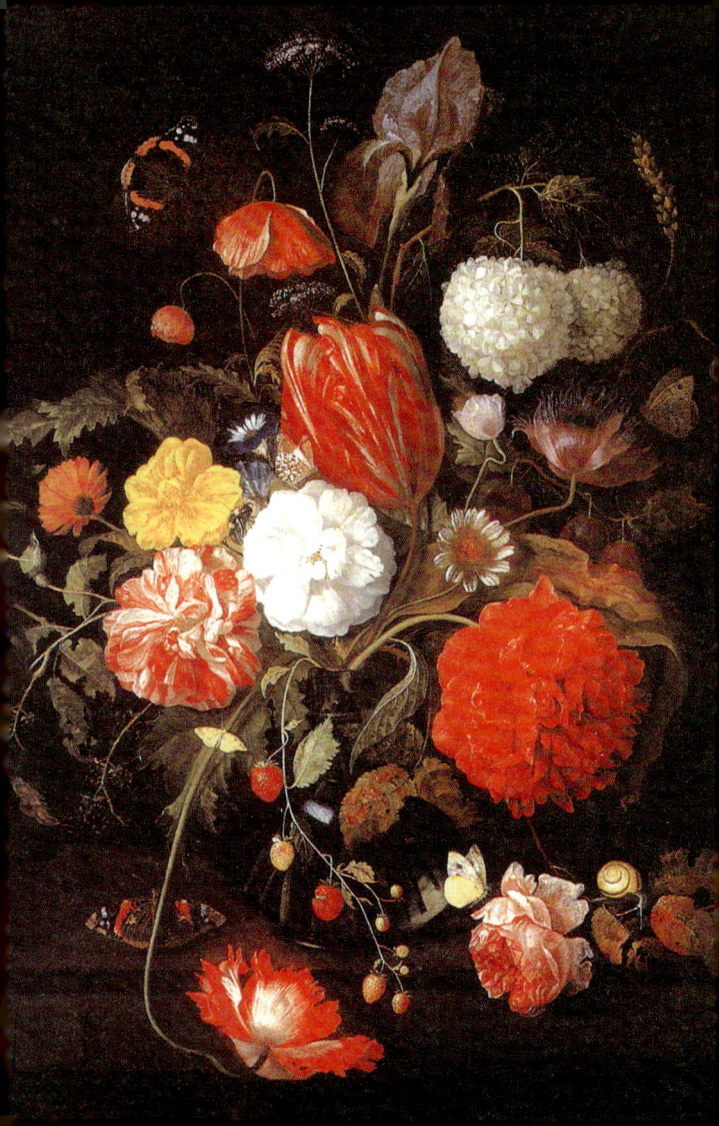

Whither Essential Oils

The **Essential Oil** is as much the **Life Force** of a Plant as the **Soul** is the Spiritual Centre of our **Being**. They Promote Growth, attract Pollinating Insects, Repel Predators and protect against disease.

Extracted, they offer us a **Rainbow of Remedies** and a **Blessing of Beauty** aids. Each oil contains hundreds of different components and although Chemists can identify each one, no Laboratory has been able to reproduce them.

Some are worth a King's Ransom. It takes the blossoms of tens of thousands of jasmine flowers to produce a few sparkling drops, each one more precious than the next. Blooms must be handpicked before dawn for Jasmine to yield its cherished oil.

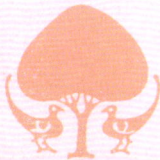

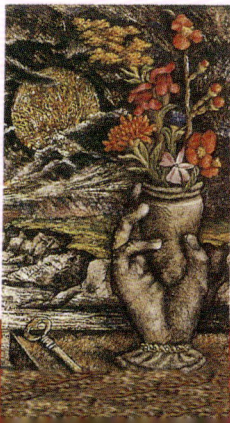

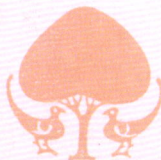

A FEW WORDS OF TECHNOLOGY

Distillation

Discovered by the Turks a thousand years ago, the Process demands that the desired part of the plant is introduced to steam or boiling water and the vapour made to journey along a network of glass tubes which forms a condenser from which the oil drops are syphoned off.

Enfleurage

The oldest and, as it can only be carried out by hand, the costliest method. The **Flower Heads** are placed on glass sheets smeared with animal fat or beeswax. Flowers are added layer upon layer until the fat is saturated with the essential oil. This **Mulch** is dissolved in alcohol which causes the fat to drop to the bottom of the container. The fluid is now heated until all the alcohol evaporates and the oil can be poured off.

Expression

Essential oils of **Citrus Fruits** are contained in tiny glands in the peel and can be obtained by crushing them, thus expressing the oil.

Solvent extraction

Flower Petals are mixed with a solvent in a huge vat and stirred for hours on end by a mechanical paddle. When the petals have been drained of their oil, the mixture is strained and the residual liquid boiled to evaporate the solvent. However, traces of the solvent linger in the oils produced by this process and they are referred to as **Absolute Oils** rather than pure **Essential Oils**.

Adieu dull technology!

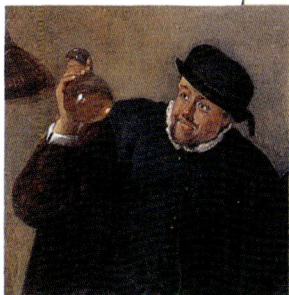

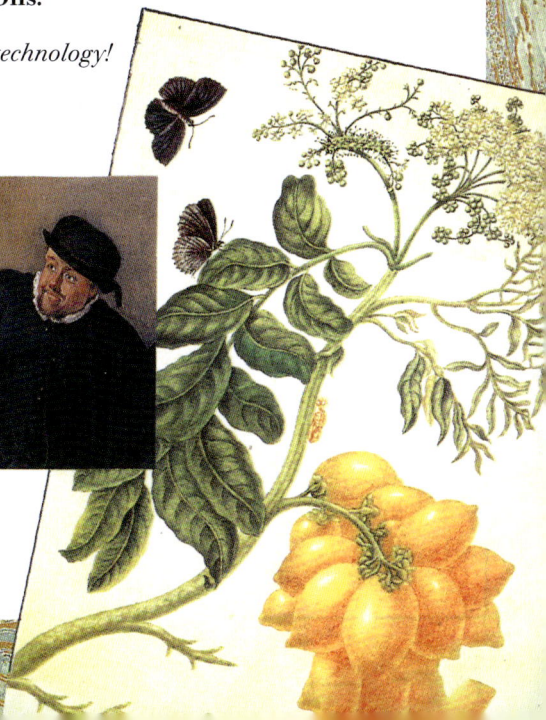

MAGICAL MIXTURES

Such is their potency that essential oils must be mixed with a **Carrier Oil** before being applied to the skin*, whether to calm an irritation brought about by being bitten by Insects or when massaged into the skin to ease aching Muscles.

Carrier or base oils are extracted from a variety of seeds such as Grapeseed, nuts which include the worthy Hazel and vegetables including Avocado, considered by many as Nature's Larder, so rich is it in nutrients.

Many of these oils, all of which are easily Absorbed into the Skin, have their own therapeutic properties, instanced here by the oil yielded by the rose-hip which is a Worthy, but alas Costly, ally for those who have had the mischance of Burning themselves.

❋ ❋ ❋

*Lavender and Tea-Tree oil are two exceptions to this rule. One or two drops of lavender oil helps remove the sting from burns, and spots and warts can safely be treated with the Modest Application, again, two drops at most, of tea tree oil.

Even in these times of Economic Stringency, it is well worth paying a Modicum Extra for unrefined, cold-pressed oils which are of Superior Benefit to their Lowly Cousins alongside whom they sit on the shelves of most Modern Purveyors of Household Aliments and Victuals.

Many of the oils hereinafter mentioned can be mixed with each other which is of Especial Use to those of Slender Means. Such admixtures allows them to benefit from the Magical Properties of some of the costlier base oils by purchasing Small Quantities of them and marrying them with an oil of Less Rank. Apricot Kernel Oil, for example, is oft a strain on the purse, but its Companionable Qualities allow it to mix well with the more affordable Almond, Grapeseed and Jojoba oils.

A helpful hint. Some expensive oils are available in more affordable capsule form. Simply pierce the capsule and release the oil captured therein by bringing Digital Pressure to bear on the capsule. That Fabled Youth-reviver **Evening Primrose** is such an oil.

Versatile if slightly Sweet **Almond Oil** is a blessing to those afflicted with dry complexions easily irritated by the Noxious Fumes that are Part and Parcel of urban life.

Such oils should be suitable for even those of the most delicate complexions, but even so it is well worth submitting oneself to a skin test lest Dame Fortune decide to frown on our oliagenous endeavours. The test is simplicity itself. Apply a dab on a part of the anatomy that is normally unseen other than by those with whom we are on intimate terms (and one which is easily accessible!). If, after two days there is no sign of any reaction, it may be safely assumed that the oil applied may be used without caution as a carrier or base oil. But even the slightest inflammation should be taken as a Warning that an allergic reaction may perchance occur if the oil is frequently and abundantly applied.

Rich **Avocado** adds youthful zest to mature skins and a glow to those who have neglected the Daily Use of a good moisturizer o'er long. It is also a staunch ally in the treatment of eczema and psoriasis, as is its kinsman, expensive **Borage**, which should be in the Armoury of All Those who refuse to let the passage of Time affect their looks to any disadvantage.

The Humble **Carrot** yields an oil that has Scar-Healing qualities, while its fellow of Yeoman Stock, the ubiquitous **Grapeseed**, light and lacking in smell, is widely available and inexpensive. It suits all skin types and is more than willing to flirt with oils of greater character to enhance its own reputation.

Light, easily absorbed but expensive **Hazelnut** is much used by those with oily or combination skins, but cheaper **Jojoba**, as light as a Summer Zephyr, is by far the best base for oils to be Smoothed into the skin.

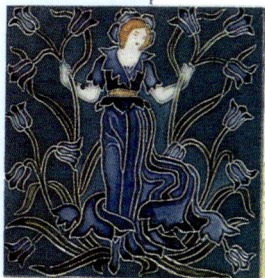

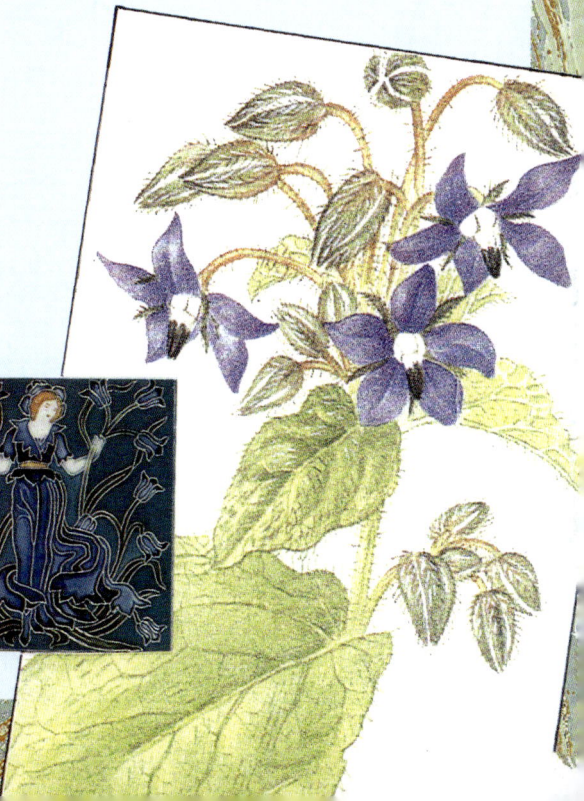

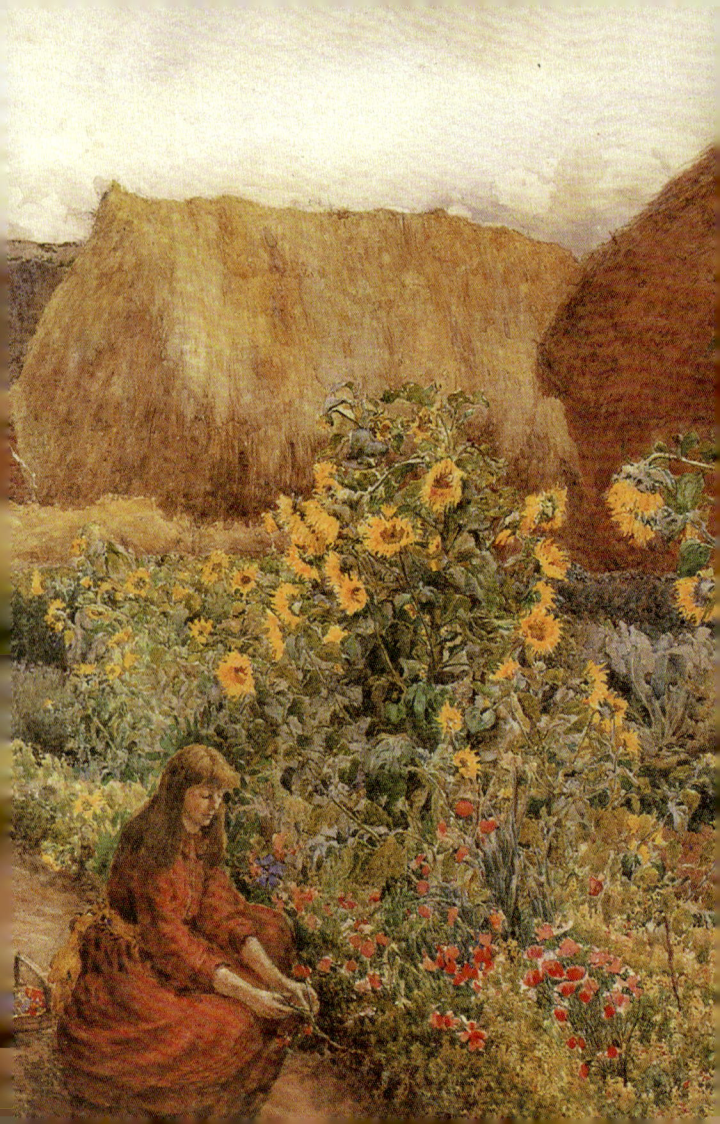

The oil yielded by the **Kukui Nut** penetrates deep into the skin and is perfect for baby, while **Macadamia Nut** oil is perfect for those at the other end of the Age Spectrum.

Despite a Strong Smell, ubiquitous **Olive Oil** is popular among those Seeking Solace for sore or dehydrated skin. **Passion-flower** oil, too, is Much Recommended as a base oil for those suffering from skin irritations or whose skin lacks elasticity, while glorious but wildly expensive **Rose Hip** is a blessing to those whose complexions have acquired a prematurely aged look.

Safflower is the star of the Bargain Basement of carrier oils: it is light and easily absorbed: she and her sister, **Sesame**, suit all skin types, as does **Sunflower** which must be used in its unrefined state.

To end this Whirlwind Walk among the Base Oils, **Walnut oil** is ideal as a carrier for a Body Massage oil as is dusky **Wheatgerm,** which is Specially Suited to those with dry skin.

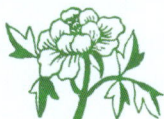

Cedarwood

The fact that much of the **Cedarwood Oil** available today is extracted from sawdust and woodshavings swept from the floors of North American cedar mills belies the noble history of this **Much-Prized** Oil and is a source of Some Confusion. The Upstart American (*Cedrus atlantica*) is all very well for use in Perfumery, but for Therapeutic Purpose, the oil of the true cedar of Moroccan Pedigree (*Cedrus libani*) must be sought out.

The Cedar tree is one of the Great Longevity. The grove of Cedars from which Wise Solomon had trees felled to build his temple, still flourishes on Mount Lebanon. Little wonder that the Egyptians held the oil yielded by these majestic trees in such awe, and used it in their medicines, cosmetics, embalming processes and burned it in their temples.

The Ancient Herbalists, Dioscorides and Galen, recorded that cedar oil prevented putrefaction, and now, two millenia later, aromatherapists are well aware that cedarwood is of much benefit in the treatment of Dermatological Complaints. To treat eczema, for example, a thrice-daily application of a tincture prepared by adding eight drops of the oil to four teaspoons of wheatgerm oil, is Highly Recommended.

True Cedarwood oil is said to have restorative powers for men whose sexual appetite has lost its Youthful Vigour: Women Wily in the Ways of aromatherapy who secrete a drop or two of cedarwood oil to lotions and potions used by their stricken menfolk for shaving or aftershaving purposes, may find this subtle subterfuge works to Mutual Satisfaction.

Members of both sexes whose hair has thinned may find the remedy detailed hereafter advantageous. Add twenty drops of true cedarwood oil to an amalgam of two tablespoonfuls of grapeseed oil and one tea-spoonful of first-pressing, virgin olive oil. The mixtures should be rubbed into the scalp and left for two hours before shampooing. Also, the addition of fifteen drops of the aforementioned oil to an average-sized bottle of a shampoo of Proprietory Nature should prove beneficial to the overall condition of the hair. (Caveat: Those who are blessed with tresses of a Fair Hue should be sparing in their use of Cedarwood Oil because of its inclination to darken the hair.)

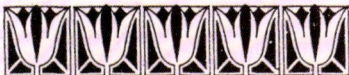

Caveat Aromatherapeutica

> I have been here before,
> But how or when I cannot tell.
> I know the grass beyond the door,
> The sweet keen smell.
>   Dante Gabriel Rosetti

While Wholeheartedly recommending the joys of **Olfactory Stimulation,** it would indeed be foolhardy to describe the ways, *which are many,* by which we can benefit from Fragrant Nature without a few timely words of caution about the Lubricants of Aromatherapy – Essential Oils.

the concentrated strength of these oils is such that it is **ill-advised** to apply them directly onto the skin. They must be diluted in a carrier oil, such as almond, before use. Furthermore they must never be ingested or taken by mouth.

save for a glass of wine at table, alcoholic beverages and essential oil therapies *do not make good companions.*

until they have been delivered of their offspring, **Ladies** who are with child must take *extra care* when using essential oils.

should, due to careless application, essential oil be introduced into the **Eye,** or that organ is found to react adversely to strong vapour, it should be bathed with cool water.

over-indulgence may have unforeseen consequences, though not, it is to be hoped, so tragic the fate that befell a guest of the **Emperor Nero.** Such was the gusto with which the unfortunate Sybarite inhaled the intensely rose-perfumed air that he succumbed to Asphyxiation and died.

those for whom Physicans have prescribed medication should refrain from the use of essential oils until their treatment has run its course.

after the application of an oil borne by any of the **Citrus Fruits** it is wise to **Seek Shade** as the aforementioned oils may irritate the skin if exposed to sunlight.

Aromatherapy's Pharmacopoeia

The shelves of **Libraries** and **Bookshops** are laden with literature concerning the **Curative Properties** of Essential Oils. In this Little Volume we can do no more than but take a whirlwind tour into Nature's Mighty Medicalia.

But few are the ailments the treatment of which can not be influenced by having resort to bountiful aromatherapy. The essential oils can be used during massage, blended into an appropriate cream, dropped into a bath, inhaled in steam, breathed deeply when used to fragrance a room with a diffuser or air freshener or dropped onto a compress.

Aches and pains vanish wonderously when treated with black pepper, chamomile, eucalyptus, frankincense, ginger, juniper, lavender, lemon, marjoram, peppermint, rosemary and thyme.

Acne can be cured by bergamot, chamomile, juniper, lavender, lemongrass, patchouli, peppermint, rosemary, sandalwood and tea-tree.

Anaemia sufferers may safely look to black pepper, chamomile, lemon, peppermint, rosemary and thyme to help normalize things.

Asthma has been known to be relieved by benzoin, cajeput, cypress, eucalyptus, frankincense, lavender, lemon, myrrh, peppermint, rosemary and thyme.

Banish **boils** with bergamot, chamomile, lavender, lemon, rosemary, tea-tree and thyme.

Benzoin, cajeput, eucalyptus, fennel, frankincense, lavender, lemon, myrrh, peppermint, rosemary, sandalwood, tea-tree and thyme are a boon to those who suffer from **bronchitis**.

Catarrh is often eased by basil, eucalyptus, black pepper, frankincense, lavender, myrrh and tea-tree. Irritating **chilblains** succumb to the charms of fragrant lemon.

Cold sores often vanish after the briefest flirtation with lavender and tea-tree while the army of allies in the treatment of **colic** includes bergamot, black pepper, chamomile, clary sage, fennel, juniper, lavender, lemongrass, marjoram and peppermint.

Colitis dislikes bergamot, black pepper, chamomile, lavender, lemongrass, neroli and rosemary.

Discomforting **constipation** is often relieved by black pepper, fennel, marjoram, rose and rosemary: **coughs** and **colds** by benzoin, black pepper, cajeput, eucalyptus, frankincense, ginger, lavender, lemon, myrrh, peppermint, rosemary, sandalwood, tea-tree and thyme: and ghastly **cystitis** by bergamot, cajeput, eucalyptus, juniper, lavender, sandalwood and tea-tree.

Banish **depression** with basil, bergamot, chamomile, clary sage, geranium, jasmine, lavender, neroli, patchouli, rose, sandalwood, tangerine, thyme and ylang-ylang.

Disturbing **dermatitis** can be cleared with benzoin, juniper, lavender, patchouli, peppermint and rosemary. A sluggish **digestive system** is often stimulated by black pepper, fennel, juniper or peppermint. Upset stomachs evidenced by **diarrhoea** may be soothed by black pepper, cajeput, chamomile, cypress, eucalyptus, rosemary and sandalwood.

Eucalpytus, geranium and juniper have proved true friends to **diabetics.**

Earache can be soothed by basil, chamomile and lavender.

Eczema crumbles against an attack by bergamot, chamomile, geranium, juniper, lavender, myrrh, patchouli and rosemary.

Fever may be treated with black pepper, chamomile, eucalyptus, ginger, juniper, lavender or peppermint. Embarrassing **flatulence** may well be calmed by bergamot, black pepper, chamomile, fennel, ginger, juniper, lavender.

Gout sufferers will find juniper, lemon, rosemary and

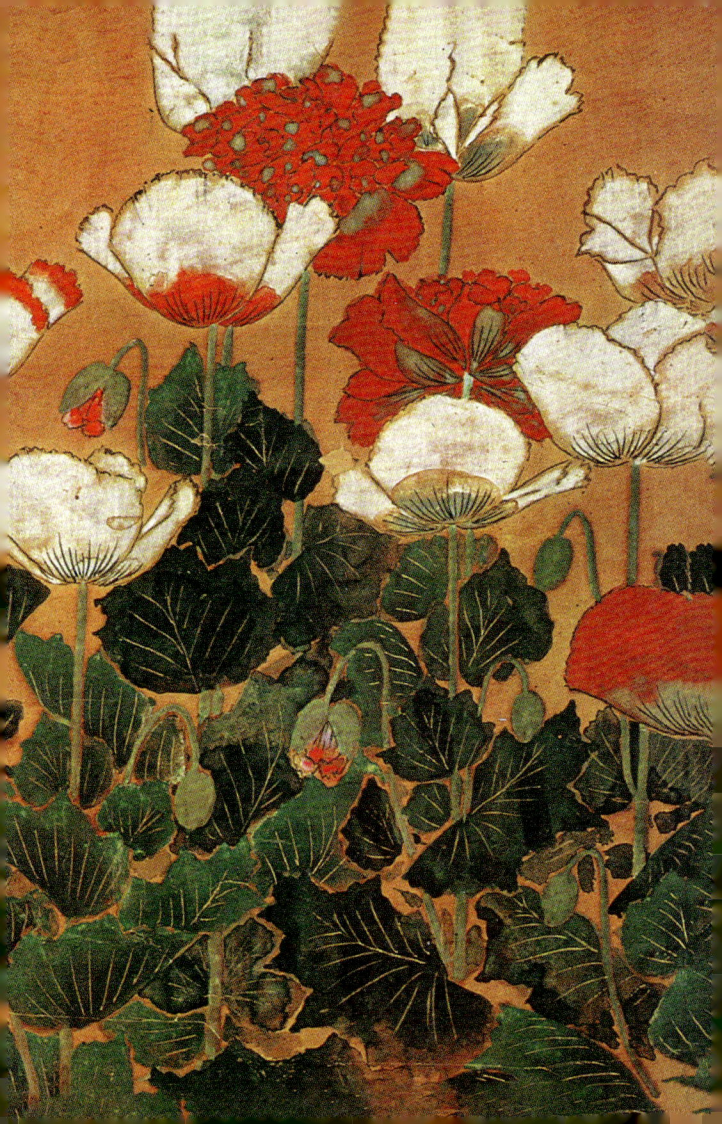

thyme ease the throbbing pain.

Fennel, juniper and rosemary are useful allies to those who have overindulged in their acquaintance with the grain or the grape and find themselves with a **hangover**. (Fennel is also used to treat those whose overfondness of liquor has led them to become dependent on it.) A **headache** of a non-alcoholic nature will be soothed by basil, chamomile, lavender, marjoram, peppermint and rosemary.

Lavender, marjoram, neroli and rose are of especial efficacy as tonic to the **heart,** while **heartburn** may be soothed by black pepper or lemon, and hiccoughs by basil, fennel or tangerine. That curse of Modern Living, **hypertension**, can be relieved by looking to Lady Chamomile and her maids-in-waiting lavender, lemon, marjoram, neroli and ylang ylang. Little sister **hypotension** can be treated with rosemary and thyme. The list of allies in the anti-**indigestion** brigade is a long one and includes basil, bergamot, chamomile, cajeput, fennel, ginger, lavender, lemongrass, marjoram, myrrh, neroli, peppermint, rosemary and tangerine.

The **liver** favours flirtation with chamomile, cypress, geranium, lavender, lemon, peppermint, rose, rosemary and tangerine.

Those who have **lost their appetite** may find their tastebuds are stimulated after a brief encounter with bergamot, black pepper, chamomile, fennel, ginger, lavender or peppermint, while those whose appetite has led them down the slippery path to **obesity** should look to fennel, juniper, lemon or rosemary to help them overcome their over-enthusiastic appetites.

Painful **neuralgia** is usually soothed by black pepper, chamomile, eucalyptus, lavender, peppermint, tea-tree and thyme.

Palpitations are often calmed by lavender, neroli, rose, rosemary and ylang-ylang, and the miseries of **Pre-Menstrual Tension** can be eased with chamomile, cypress, geranium, lavender and rose.

Tonsilitis succumbs to attention from benzoin, cajeput, eucalyptus, geranium, ginger, lavender, lemon and sandalwood.

Chamomile and peppermint can help to relieve the enervating pain of **toothache.** Those afflicted by **travel sickness** should look to ginger or peppermint for relief.

It should be, of course, unnecessary to advise that if any symptom lingers for more than a day or two, the advice of a qualified physician should be sought . . .

CHAMOMILE

So-called from the Greek for Earth Apple, because of its apple-like smell. It is a composite plant, the flowers of which are used in Medicine for their bitter and tonic properties.

The list of ailments which are reputed to benefit from *Anthemis noblis* and her sister *Matricaria recutita* ranges from colitis to rheumatism. Young men and women cursed with the dreaded acne should resort to this powerful essence, as should anyone suffering from anxiety, boils, chilblains, colic, colitis, herpes, indigestion, insomnia and a host of other complaints.

Chamomile harmonizes, soothes and pacifies. Those who sing its praises loudest advocate its use for the sweet serenity with which it imbues them. Those who have advocated its use in the past include the sagacious Hippocrates who dedicated it to the Sun because 'it cures the ague'. In 1656, that worthiest of herbalists, John Parkinson, wrote that a bath whose waters were rich in Chamomile could be used 'to comfort and strengthen the sound and ease the pain in the diseased.'

Those who yearn for a night wrapped in Morpheus's welcoming embrace should find that a few drops of Chamomile oil added to their evening bath will encourage this oft-elusive God of Slumber to call.

Anyone coping with grief occasioned by the passing of a Loved One may find chamomile a solace during their darkest hours. While those whose overfondness for the bottle has led them into the terrifying arms of *Delirium Tremens* should seek out noble chamomile whose staunch friendship will lead them back to the light.

Noble it may be, but Chamomile's Lofty Station does not prevent her from blending happily with geranium, lavender, rose and ylang ylang oils.

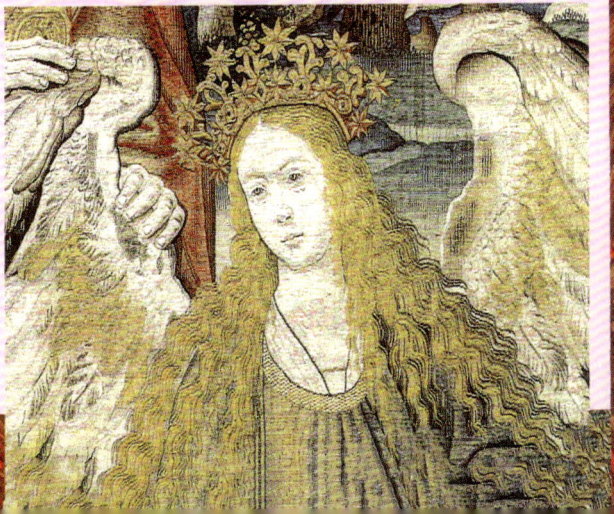

PERSONALITY POINTERS

The **Essential Oils** you favour can tell you a lot about your personality. If you like the floral oils you tend to be **Dynamic and Confident** *whereas* if you prefer the oils extracted from leaves you can be **Melancholic and Detached.** Choose one from the following eight oils and judge for yourself how your nose points to your personality.

Bergamot-Clary Sage-Patchouli Frankincense Ginger-Dill-Cardamom-Cedarwood

If **Bergamot** tantalized your olfactory glands you are engaging, reliable, companionable, bright and benevolent, although you can be indecisive, defensive, insecure, anxious and immature.

Those who chose **Clary Sage** are loving and generous, welcoming and supportive with a tendency to be manipulative, domineering, and something of a hypochondriac.

Those who preferred **Patchouli** are wise and creative, rejuvenating and understanding, cynical, hostile, mean and over critical.

Fans of **Frankincense** have the wisdom of Solomon but the pride of a muster of peacocks, the ethics of a saint but the intolerance of Herod.

Those who had **Ginger** at the top of their list have the patience of Job and the loyalty of Lassie; sadly, they tend to be as absent minded as the proverbial professor, with the get-up-and-go of an over-dressed lettuce leaf.

Devotees of **Dill** have the energy of a puppy and the intuition of a telepath, but their fits of melancholy and their aloof nature can put others off.

Oh Happy **Cardamom.** Sophisticated high-fliers, extrovert entrepreneurs; no wonder colleagues find you superficial, impolite, ill-mannered and occasionally debauched!

Self-reliance is the key word for **Cedar-woodians:** assertive, earnest and steadfast. Who would have thought that these pinnacles of perfection include Ivan the Terrible and Ebeneezer Scrooge.

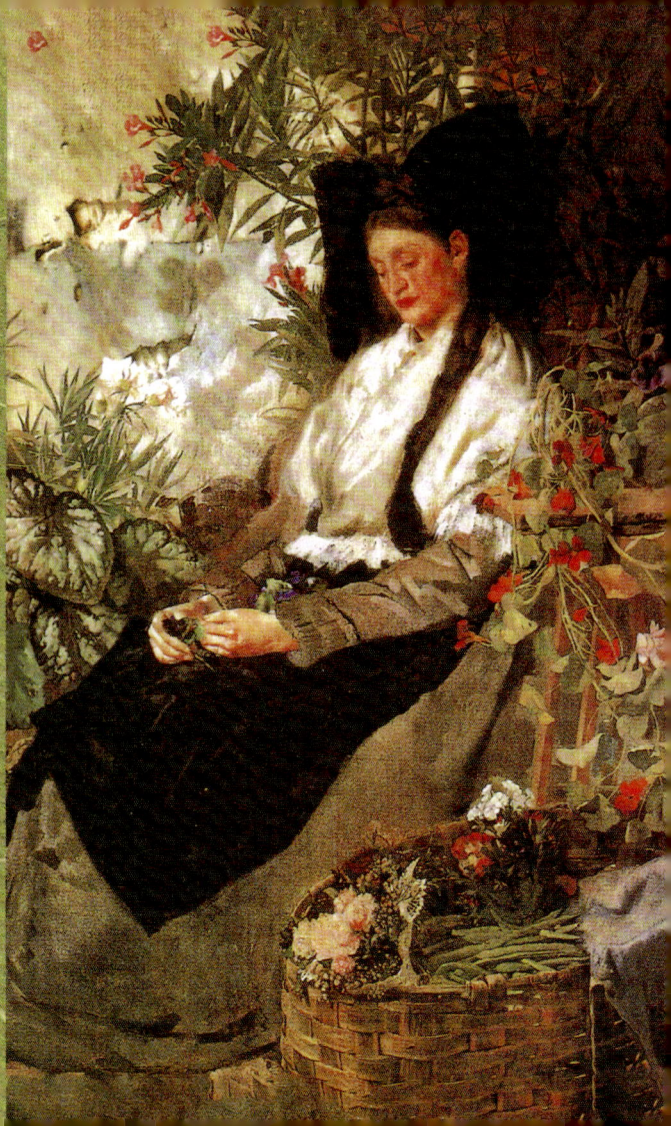

FLOWER POWER

We all go through periods when **Life Gets Us Down.** Uncertainty in the **Workplace** may lead to **Tensions** in the **Home**: a **Relationship** may not be going as smoothly as we would wish: something, we know not what, seems to be holding us back from reaching our true potential. And often these Cares and Concerns reveal themselves in the form of a Malady of some sort.

If these words worry you over much, **Fear Not**, for whatever the problem, help is at hand in the form of **Edward Bach** and his **Most Marvellous Flower Remedies.**

Mr. Bach was born near Birmingham in 1886 and after gaining his medical qualifications spent several years investigating the role of bacteriology in Chronic Disease before setting up a lucrative practice in London.

The more he treated the rich and stylish who flocked to his door, the more he became convinced that his patients' personalities not only affected their symptoms, but also the way they responded to treatment. This led him to coin his oft-repeated axiom, 'Take No Notice of the Disease, think only of the Personality of the One in Distress.' Illness, he proposed, was a **Distress**

Signal fired by our inner being calling for a change in our way of living and our mental outlook.

It was not to conventional medicine that he turned, but to the **Plant Kingdom** at first in the form of **Homeopathy** and later with his **Flower Remedies.** In 1930 he rejected fashionable Harley Street and repaired to the countryside where he rambled hither and yon gathering the plants and flowers which, he believed, held the key to **Health** and **Happines**.

The Good Doctor found 38 flowers that covered all known negative states of mind. These pestilants of the psyche he categorized under seven major headings: those for **Apprehension,** for **Uncertainty** and **Indecision,** for **Lack of Interest in Present Circumstances,** for **Over-sensitiveness to Ideas and Influence**, for **Despondence and Despair**, and for **Over-care in the Welfare of Others**.

He was skilled at inducing in himself the negative state of mind for which a cure was needed and then meandering through the countryside until he was 'led' to find the flowers that would immediately restore **Harmony** and **Serenity** and, within a few hours, banish any Physical Manifestations of the **Negativity.**

The Remedies themselves are readily available in Discerning Pharmacies, but better, how much better, to follow the Good Doctor's example and search the countryside for the plants and flowers we need preparatory to making our own tinctures.

There are three stages in the preparation of the remedies – making the Mother Tincture, the preparation of the Stock Bottle, and the making of the Treatment bottle.

The **Mother Tincture** is prepared by one of two methods, the simplest of which the **Sun Method** is appropriate for flowers that bloom in late spring and in the summer when the sun is at the height of its power. The necessary flowers are gathered with the **Greatest Tenderness** at about nine o'clock in the morning, by which time the freshly opened blooms will be at their most perfect, having **Bathed in Sunshine** for some hours. The flowers are put in a bowl filled with springwater and placed in strong sunlight for three hours. Miracles are afoot as the energy from the blooms is transferred to the water.

The second method entails boiling: flowers and twigs are again garnered at nine o'clock, but are simmered in springwater for half an hour before being drained.

To prepare the **Stock Bottle**, **Mother Tincture** is introduced to a Little Brandy which acts as a preservative. The spiritous admixture is now put into a sealable bottle which should then be labelled with the name of the remedy and the word 'stock'.

The Treatment Bottles contain precious drops of the liquid from the stock bottle mixed with pure spring-water and a little brandy. It is to this bottle that we resort when we seek remedy from whatever ails us.

To take the remedy, add two drops from the Treatment bottle to a glass of natural mineral water or fruit juice and take a sip every five minutes until the mood subsides. Hold the water in the mouth for a few moments and as you swallow picture it as a cleansing light illuminating the whole system, dazzling the unwanted condition out of existence.

One or two drops from an appropriate **Floral Remedy Stock Bottle** can be added to massage oil to most beneficial advantage, and the effects of a traditional **Aromatherapy Bath** can be enhanced by five or six drops of a suitable **Floral Remedy.**

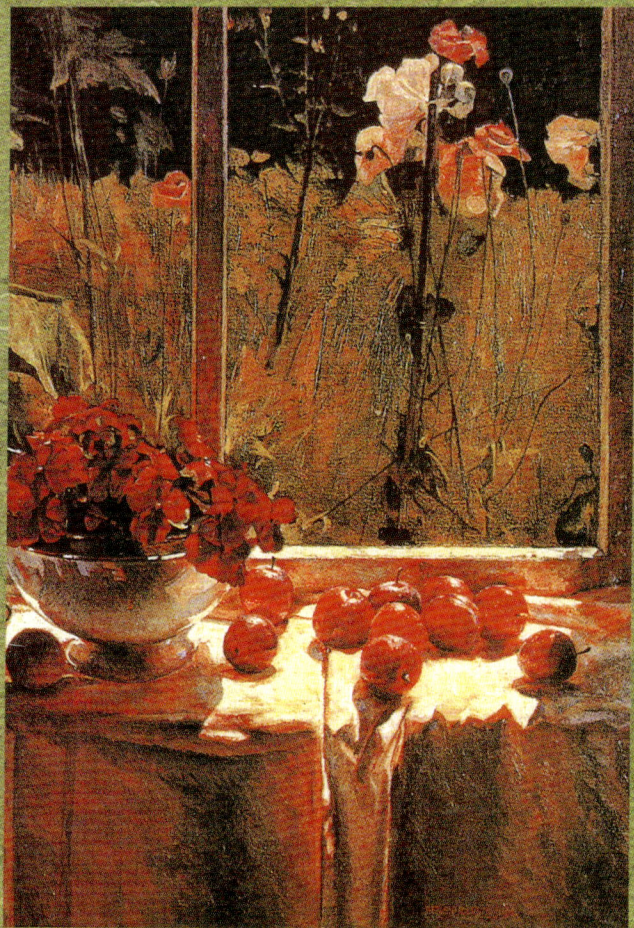

Thirty-eight Miracles

Dr Bach identified thirty-eight healers from the world of nature to counter the negativity that manifests itself in ill health. These natural miracle-makers range from delicate Cherry Plum blossoms to Hearty Heather, from Fragrant Honeysuckle to Mighty Elm. In affirming their Most Perfect Properties, Dr Bach wove common sense with Uncommon Wisdom as we can perceive when reading his Musings on Mimulus:

Fear in reality holds no place in the natural kingdom, since the Divinity within us, which is ourself, is unconquerable and immortal, and if we could but realize it we, as Children of God, have nothing of which to be afraid.

Agrimony helps those who hide their inner heartache behind a happy-go-lucky exterior to realize that letting-go is not weakness but a sign of True Strength.
Aspen is Most Efficacious for those moments when we are overcome by an impending Sense of Doom, dreadful moments to which we are all at sometime prone.
Beech replaces intolerance with tolerance, adds approval where there was criticism and exchanges Arrogance for Humility.

Cerato encourages those who have No Confidence in their own judgment to act without always seeking the approval of others.

Cherry Plum is a boon to people who, for whatever reason, fear for their own Mental Well-being.

Chestnut Bud helps people who fail to Learn from Past Mistakes so to do.

Chicory discourages attention-seeking, over-possessiveness and self-pity.

Clematis brings the dreamy who lack interest in the present down to earth, not with a bang, but with Gentle Encouragement.

Crab Apple helps overcome self-hatred and helps those bogged down with heavy thoughts. It is the only Floral Remedy prescribed for physical complaints, namely, Acne, Eczema and Psoriasis.

Elm restores confidence in those who feel Overburdened by Responsibility.

Gentian puts heart into those who are too Easily Discouraged.

Gorse helps anyone who has come to the end of the road and views the future with hopeless despair not to give up, that there is Light at the End of the Tunnel.

Heather encourages those obsessed with their own troubles to lend a sympathetic ear to Others.

Holly copes with the prickly subjects of Hatred, Jealousy and Envy.

Honeysuckle helps those who live in the past to Waken up to the Present.

Hornbeam banishes that weary Monday-morning feeling and puts a Spring in the Step.

Impatiens, as its name suggests, soothes the impatient of this world, and makes the irritable Less So.

Larch banishes lack of confidence and inferiority complexes. It helps those who always anticipate failure to face the Future with Confidence.

Mimulus helps those stricken by fear of the Unknown.

Mustard sends Black Depression on its way.

Oak is for those who struggle against all odds and who feel despondent at the prospect of yet more Struggle, Struggle, Struggle.

Olive boosts energy levels, physical and mental, and is beneficial to those Recovering from Illness.

Pine helps those who constantly reproach themselves, taking the blame for the mistakes of others.

Red Chestnut is to be recommended for those generous people who are fearful or over-concerned for the Welfare of Others.

Rock Rose treats Fear, Terror and Panic most benignly.

Star of Bethlehem calms those suffering from the long term effect of shock - be it the drama of a car crash or the Trauma of Bereavement.

Sweet Chestnut helps those who believe there is no tomorrow to realize that there *will* be a new dawn, and that they will be there to Glory in its Soft Light.

Vervain puts over-enthusiasm in its place.

Vine makes the domineering more flexible and those who strive for power less Ruthless in its Pursuit.

Walnut helps people adapt to change, from women with menstrual problems to babies with teething pains.

Water Violet encourages humility in the proud and makes the burden of Loneliness more easy to bear.

White Chestnut encourages Morpheus to visit those who lie awake at night plagued by unwanted thoughts.

Wild Oat, well sown, is for people who are uncertain that they are treading the right path in life, whose choice of career has left them Bored and Frustrated.

Wild Rose rouses the Apathetic who are resigned to their lot and make no attempt to improve things.

Willow dries the eyes of those who shed bitter tears of Resentment.

GERANIUM

Those seeking geranium oil of Superior Quality should look to the island of Reunion or to Egypt where climate and soil quality combine to produce Perfect Pelargonia of the seven species that give us geranium oil. It takes over one thousand pounds weight of the plant, which must be freshly cut just before the flowers open, to yield just two pounds of the oil. While not too expensive, the oil may be beyond the means of many, especially in these days of Economic Uncertainty. Fear not, for it mixes well with other, cheaper, oils.

Its balancing properties make it popular for aromatherapy massage, and is a valuable ally in the struggle against unsightly accumulations of the dreaded cellulite. And at the risk of Appearing Indelicate, those afflicted by painful haemorrhoids may seek relief by adding a single drop of Geranium oil to a small jar of cold cream and, in the privacy of the bathroom, applying the cream to the Afflicted Part.

Sufferers from Athlete's Foot should bathe the Feet in warm water mixed with sea salt and five drops of geranium oil. Then Massage with three drops each of wheatgerm and geranium oils in a soya oil base. Repeat twice daily and the Frightful Fungus will Fade.

To create a suitable ambience for an intimate *diner à deux,* drop equal quantities of geranium, bergamot and lavender with a *soupçon* of cinnamon bark into a saucer set atop a radiator. The aroma given off is as subtle as it is seductive. The oil on its own, similarly positioned, is a wonderful pick-me-up, especially for those whose lot it is to study late into the night, and five drops mixed with two teaspoonsfuls of soya oil and massaged into the temples, sinus area, the backs of the neck and hands and clockwise into the solar plexus is a Perfect Pick-You-Up, especially if you lie down for five minutes after your brief *sortie* into the world of self-massage.

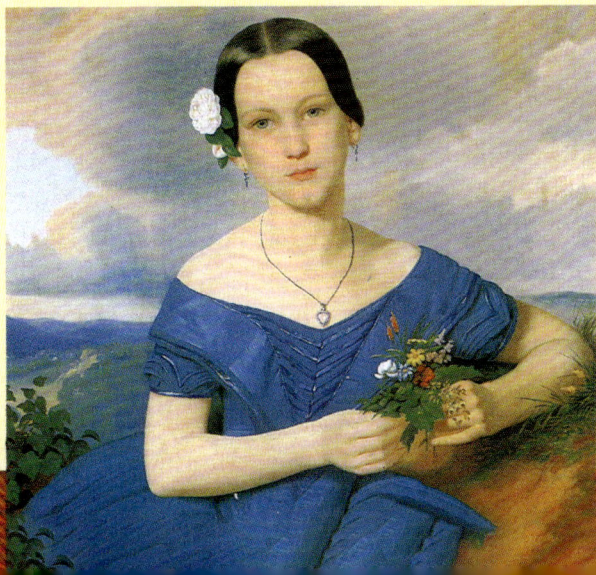

GINGER

The rhizomes of the plant *Zingibe officinale,* a native of China, yield an oil which, though not as intensely aromatic as the root of the plant when freshly ground, is still strong enough to dominate when blended with other oils.

Its strength is such that it must never be rubbed directly onto the skin or added undiluted to a bath: and in any concentration it is unsuitable for those with sensitive skins and for women who are with child.

This **Scintillating Spice** has much that is praiseworthy. The Ancient Eygptians used it to ward off threatening epidemics: the Greeks held that it stimulated the digestion system, while the Romans used it as part of a preparation which was efficacious in the treatment of cataracts of the Eye.

St Hildegarde, the twelfth-century healer, credited ginger with stimulatory powers of a sexual nature, especially useful for men of a Certain Age. The receipt credited to the Saintly Woman (but which may, perhaps, be of much Earlier Origin) was one part oil of rosemary mixed with two parts each of savory and clove oils, three of wheatgerm and ginger, the whole added to an

Appropriate Amount of soya oil and massaged onto the nether regions of the spine. The patient was then administered of a tisane of grated ginger dissolved in hot water along with a pinch of rosemary and a pinch of savory: a stick of cinnamon was added to the liquid for five minutes, after which the tisane was Partaken Of.

Ginger has been used successfully (albeit with care) in the treatment of arthritis, chilblains, nervous tension and to the benefit of those suffering from colds, cramp, fibrositis, poor circulation and rheumatism.

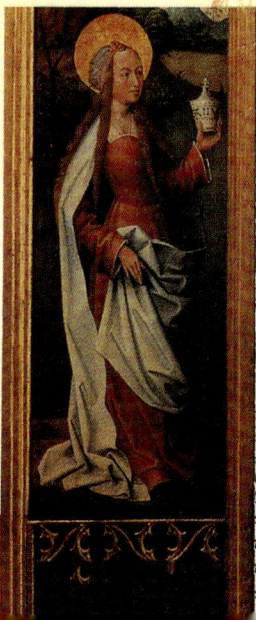

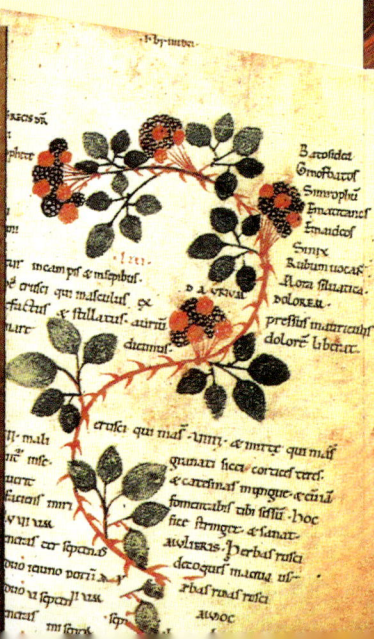

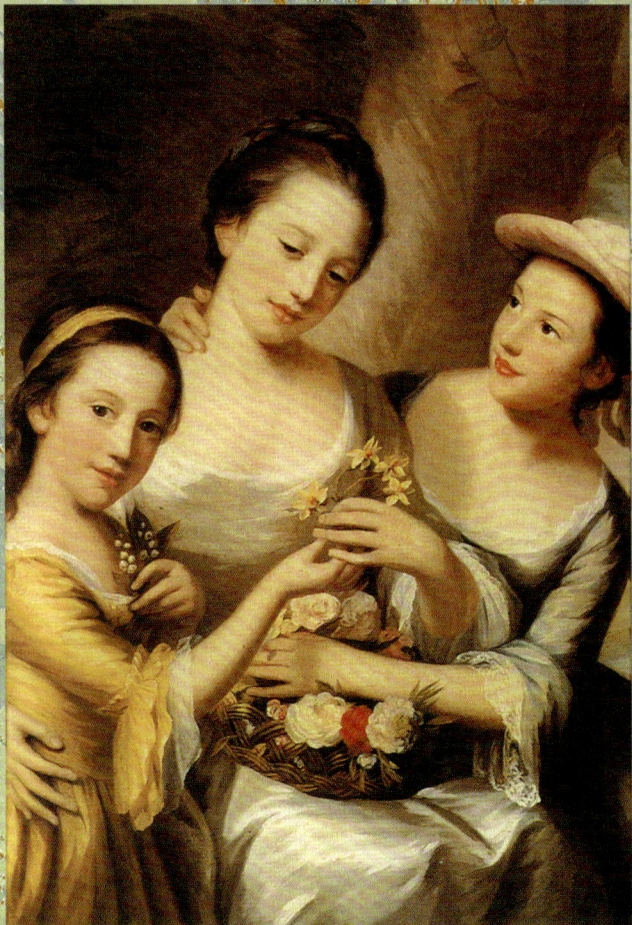

A Flawless Complexion

Fortunate are those endowed with smooth, blemish-free skin, not too oily, not too dry. Those who cannot be counted among that happy few can rummage among Aromatherapy's *largesse* of lotions to solve problematic skin conditions.

Those for whom **youth** is but a rose-tinted memory should look to Friendly Frankincese, Loyal Lavender, Mysterious Myrrh, Sprightly Sandalwood for help. Dehydrated skins succumb to Captivating Chamomile, Generous Geranium, the ever-faithful Lady Lavender and Regal Rose.

For all skins except the most delicate a tincture of Lavender, Geranium, Jojoba and Almond regularly applied will soon show its benefits. Those whose skin is on the **dry side** should massage into a thoroughly cleansed skin a mixture of Avocado oil, Peach-nut oil and Wheatgerm Oil into which some drops of Geranium and Rose oil have been added. Ladies can say goodbye to oily skin by applying Ylang-Ylang, Lemon, Cypress and Petitgrain mixed with Grapeseed Oil, while those with problem skins should look to a mixture of Myrrh and Chamomile, Bois de Rose and Lavender in Kukui nut oil for relief.

Relief for those who have ignored **Current Medical Advice** and worshipped too long at the **Temple of Helios**; a lotion of Lavender in Avocado oil applied to the sunbruised area several times a day. Those of greater wisdom who seek the shade during sunny spells but who find the heat uncomfortable can cool themselves with a refreshing spray from a bottle containing Sparkling Mineral Water to which two drops of Peppermint and three of Neroli have been added. The self-same spray is a great favourite with many women whose lifestyle necessitates frequent travel by aeroplane.

Essential oils can also be used in the preparation of skin creams such as this extremely efficacious lotion. To make it melt ¾oz (15gr) of grated beeswax in 2 fluid ounces (56ml) Jojoba and 3 fluid ounces (84ml) Almond oil in a heat-proof basin over a saucepan of simmering water. While the wax is melting into the oils, heat 1 fluid ounce (28ml) of distilled water in similar fashion until it is about blood heat. Add the water drop by drop to the melting mixture, beating with a whisk or electric food mixer set at medium fashion after each drop has been added. Continue in similar fashion until two teaspoonfuls of the water have been used at which point remove the pan from the heat and continue as before until all the water has been used. As soon as the mixture thickens, stir in six to eight drops of the chosen essential oil and divide the mixture into sterilized pots of suitable size and cover tightly.

Not only does the aforementioned method give you the freedom to select the oils you wish, it is also easier on the purse than the expensive creams we are exorted to purchase in the perfume halls of high street emporia.

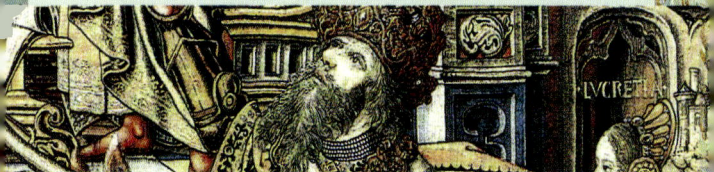

And a word for Men Folk. When Shaving, the razor blade exfoliates the skin as well as removing the daily growth. That said, there is no need for complacency. Aromatherapy is not a domain exclusive to the Fair Sex. Its bounty is there for all to enjoy. There are spice fragrances; woody ones; scents as masculine as a Pugilist's Perspiration. So why not select one, or an agreeable blend and make an after-shave lotion that will be exclusively yours by simply adding a few drops of your chosen oil to distilled water containing a dash of cider vinegar. Shake well and, *Hey Presto*, Flower Power will soothe just-shaved skin.

FRANKINCENSE & MYRRH

Frankincense was one of the three gifts brought by the Magi to the Christ Child. Tradition has it that it was carried by King Caspar. It was valued as much as gold and, along with Myrrh, was widely traded.

Frankincense is extracted from the hardened Resin of the tree *Boswellia thurifa*, appearing as tear-shaped drops on the trunk. The aroma of Frankincense when heated is oily and resinous, redolent of Pines. It has been proved that it contains the slightly Addictive Drug trihydrocannabonile. The aromatic vapour deepens the breathing, which in turn Calms the Mind. It is this particular quality which makes it an effective Aid to Meditation and Relaxation. Its use in churches creates an atmosphere condusive to Prayer. It has been reported that Altar Boys regularly exposed to Incense can form a mild dependency to it.

Inextricably linked with **Myrrh** it mixes most effectively with it for Great Therapeutic Effect. It is helpful when used to relieve problems of the Respiratory Tract such as Coughs and Catarrh, as well as Nosebleeds.

Skin troubles ranging from Acne and Oily Skin to Age-ing Skin can be alleviated when Frankincense is blend-ed with Lavender, Myrrh and Sandalwood. Other essen-tial oils which enhance the properties of Frankincense include Basil and Coriander.

Readers who have discovered that Meditation or Yoga helps them to cope with the Stresses and Strains of modern life, will find that the aroma exuded by a few drops of Frankincense in a dish of hot water concen-trates the mind most wondrously.

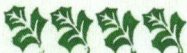

After the birth of Our Lord '. . . they presented unto him gifts: Gold and Frankincense and Myrrh.' And after His crucifixion: '. . . there came also Nicodemus, which at first came to Jesus by night and brought a mixture of Myrrh and Aloes, about an hundred pounds weight.'

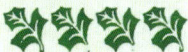

How the Oil yielded by a Sturdy Little Bush growing in Africa and Araby came to be esteemed so, is lost in the Mists of Time, but the properties ascribed to Mys-tical Myrrh have been recorded for over 3,700 years. It was well known to the Ancient Egyptians who used it in

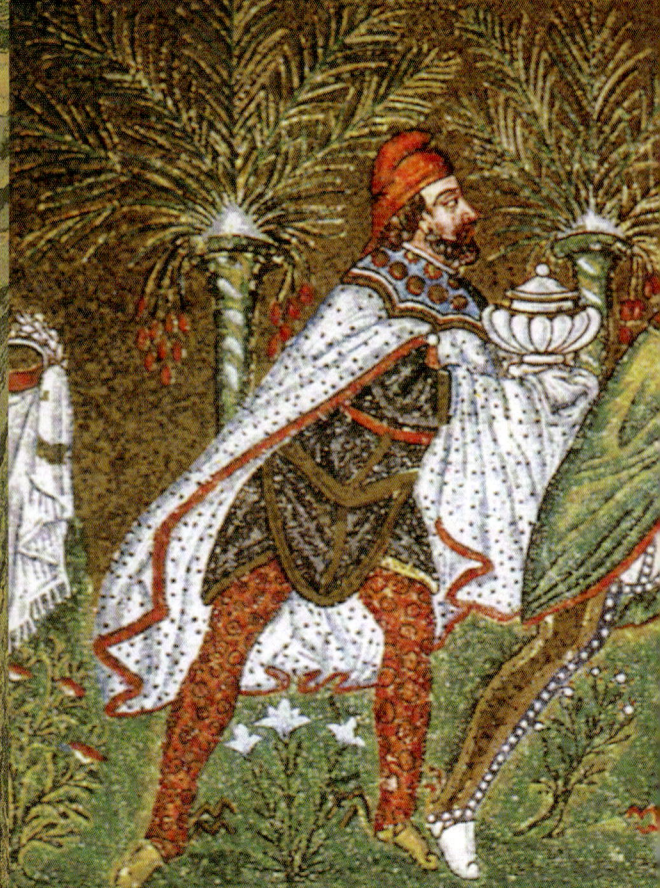

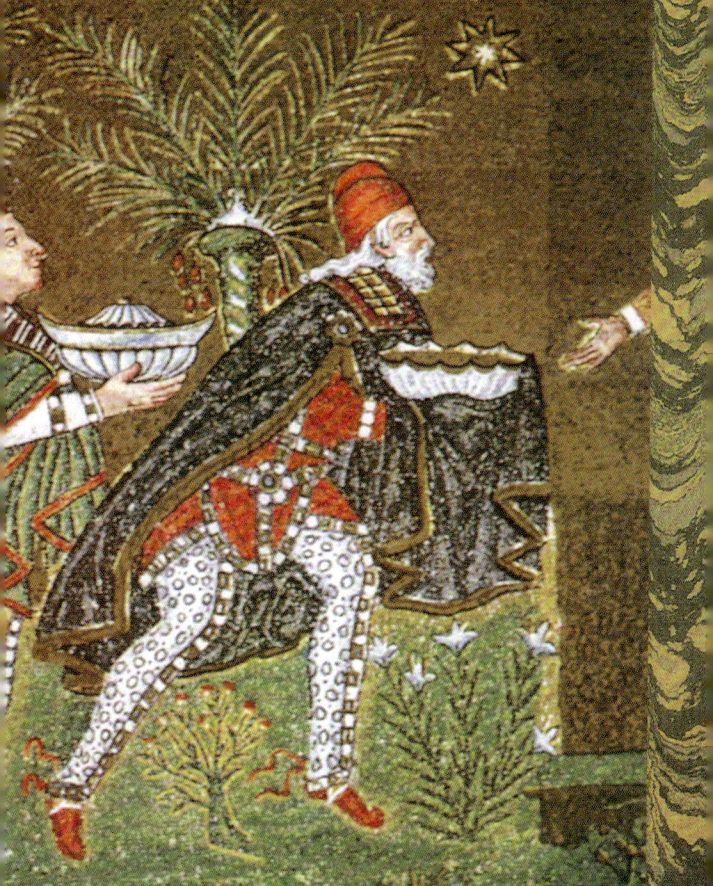

MELCHIOR ✠ SCS GASPAR

their Embalming processes and as a cure for Hay Fever. When the Children of Israel were led out of Egypt, they took with them flasks of Myrrh to use in their Religious Ceremonies.

We can deduce that Myrrh was widely used in Roman times for it is recorded in the annals of that city that in the 1st century AD, between 450 and 600 tons of Myrrh were delivered from Arabia.

Myrrh, with its spicy, slightly musty aroma so redolent of Balsam has long been used to relieve catarrh, chronic bronchitis and other complaints of the chest. It stimulates the digestive tract and relieves Flatulence.

Gargling with water to which two drops of oil of Myrrh (or one of Myrrh and one of Mint or Cardamom) have been added, is an excellent treatment for disorders of the Mouth and Gums such as gingivitis, mouth ulcers and pyorrhoea. It should not, though, be swallowed.

A mixture of ten drops each of oils of Myrrh, Palmarose and Frankincense, and one tablespoon of both Borage and Flaxseed oil is a boon for those afflicted with Skin Problems.

Myrrh is a compliant partner with several other oils, blending well with Cedarwood, the Citrus essences, Cypress, Frankincense, Juniper, Neroli, Patchouli, Petitgrain, Rose, Sandalwood and Vetiver.

The not inconsiderable cost of Oil of Myrrh may discourage its use by the more parsimonious among us. But they may still benefit from it by grinding Myrrh Resin or powder (available from better Apothecaries) in a Mortar or a Mechanical Grinder used exclusively for aromatherapy. The powder should then be mixed with a carrier oil and allowed to Rest for a Few Days before Use.

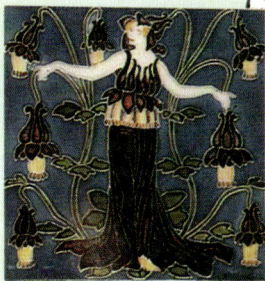

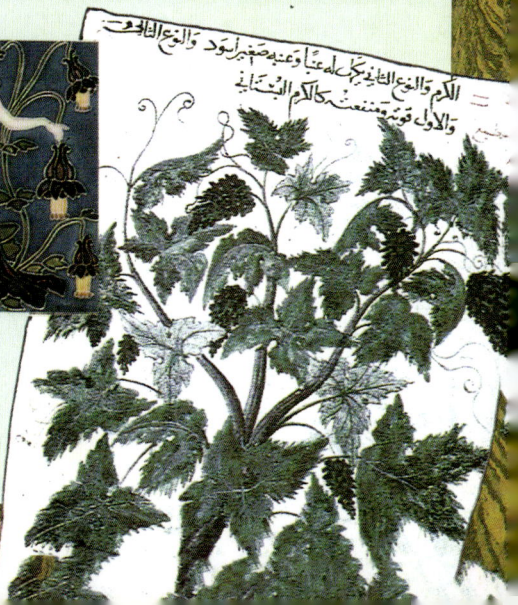

GLORIOUS TRESSES

Since **Plutarch** wrote that a fine head of hair adds beauty to a good face, many men have looked to Polyhymnia for inspiration when writing about woman's crowning glory. Milton mentions hair that 'shone like a meteor streaming into the wind.' And when Richard Lovelace in his prison cell lay on his narrow pallet and thought of his true-love, Althea, he saw himself lying 'tangled in her hair'.

The following admixtures will help promote **Natural Sheen.** One teaspoonful should be massaged into the scalp, and left for a few hours to allow the oils to penetrate before being washed off. Better to apply the oil, swathe the head in a towel and retire to bed for the night. Thrice weekly applications are recommended until the hair is aglow with good health.

For those blessed with Normal Hair two tablespoons of Jojoba oil to which eight drops of Thyme, six each of Sage and Chamomile and five of Lavender have been added makes an excellent and not too costly lotion. Or, a similar amount of Jojoba combined with eight drops each of Cedarwood, Rosemary and Sweet Bay, and three of Geranium is equally good.

Those who suffer from Dry Hair should find that the application of a blend of ten drops each of Sandalwood and Bois de Rose, five of Palmarosa and two tablespoons of Jojoba restores life and lustre to their hair.

Anyone with overactive sebaceous glands *and,* as a result, oily hair, will find that eight drops each of Petitgrain, Lemon and Lavender mixed into two tablespoons of Hazelnut oil make an exceedingly good remedy.

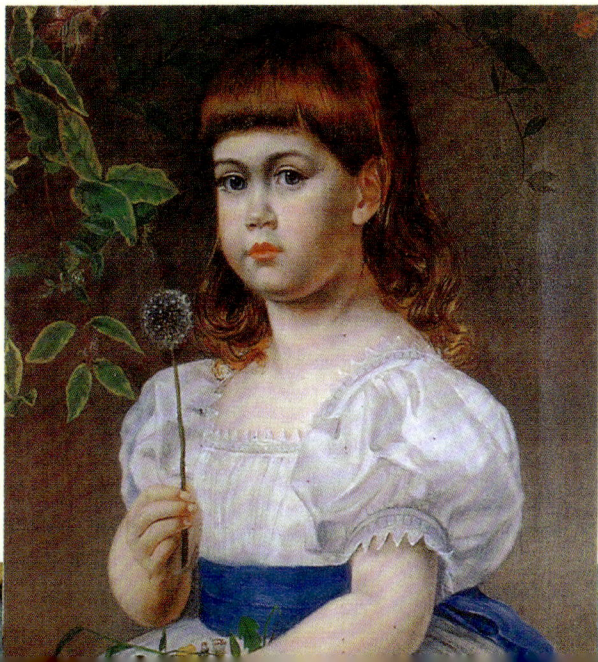

LAVENDER

That lavender has long been used to perfume bathwater is evidenced by its very name which comes from the Latin, *lavare* which means 'to wash', but it is more, so much more, than just the gentle fragrance so beloved of elderly members of the fair sex.

Gentle lavender is a **Bountiful Balancer** of **Remarkable Ability**, calming and soothing, stimulating and invigorating, according to the body's needs. Applied neat to the skin it encourages burns to heal with the Utmost Alacrity.

The list of agues and complaints that can be treated by doughty lavender ranges from abscesses and acne to migraines and muscular pains.

A few drops of lavender oil added to one's bathwater is said to help decrease horrible cellulite, while two drops added to the final rinse after shampooing the hair is to be recommended for those whose overactive sebaceous glands give their tresses an oily texture.

French lavender pickers evidenced their crop's remarkable talent for curing headaches by tucking a sprig under their hats, while Charles VI who ruled that fair land during the time of Agincourt insisted that his pillows and cushions be stuffed with the fragrant shrub. The fact that he lost to Henry V of England at the Aforementioned battle, was known as Charles the Foolish and died insane, is no reflection on his liking of lavender!

Lavender bags have, for centuries, been found in linen folds and wardrobes to gently fragrance the bedding and clothes stored therein.

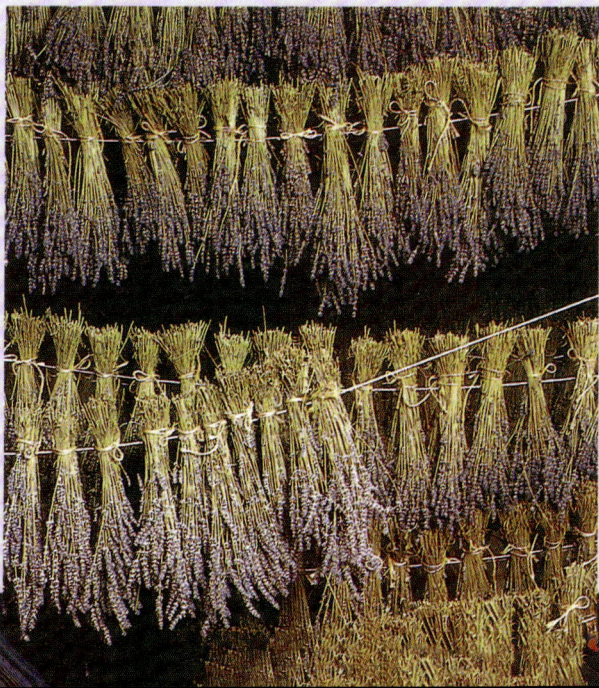

THE PARFUMIER'S ART

Little wonder that *Maître de Parfum* Marcel Rochas remarked: 'One is aware of a woman's perfume before one sees her . . . her perfume creates the first impression. If I do not know her, I can imagine her. If I do know her, it is a lovely reminder.'

It was by Lingering in the Smoke of a Fire in which a scattering of fragrant leaves and petals were smouldering that men and women first scented their bodies. Hence the word 'perfume' which literally means 'through smoke'.

Apollonia of Herophila in his *Treatise on Perfume* wrote 'Perfumes smell sweetest when the scent comes from the wrist'. That chicest of chic creatures, Coco Chanel, demurred: she advised women to wear perfume where they intended to be kissed.

Using perfume to optimum effect is a subtle skill. Those for whom the same fragrance satisfies throughout the day should, as a postscript to the morning *toilette* and with Madame Chanel's advice in mind, apply a light *eau de toilette* of the fragrance to the desired places and repeat the application mid-morning. After luncheon, and again in the evening while dressing for dinner, a few drops of the more concentrated *extrait* of the same perfume intensifies the aroma.

The woman (and in these fast, Modern Times, the male of the species, too) who wishes to present a different, perhaps richer, more sophisticated scent to the world after nightfall should ensure that it comes from the same *perfumier* as worn earlier; perfumes from the same house usually mix in *Happy Harmony*.

A worldly woman of the Author's acquaintance is never without soap scented with the perfume she favours in her portmanteau. By applying her chosen *eau de toilette* in the morning and using the ever-present tablet whenever she needs to wash her hands, she thus maintains her fragrant self from morning to night.

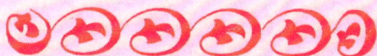

The woman who wishes to distance herself from the Gust of **Proprietary Perfumes**, need look no further than the richly aromatic shelves of the aromatherapist's larder.

The receipts are legion. Here are one as innocent as a Maiden Aunt, the other as seductive as the Enchantress after whom it is named.

Victorian Violet

When wearing this delightful but delicate scent, it is easy to imagine that you have drifted into a country cottage garden. Into a quarter-ounce mixing bottle, drizzle one part (four drops) oil of Lilac, one part Juniper, two parts Vetiver, three parts Heliotrope and ten of Violet. Fill the bottle with a commercial diluent, though not brimfully so, seal and turn it caressingly in the hand for a moment or two to encourage consummation of the marriage of the Various Oils. Transfer the perfume to an elaborate, darkly coloured bottle, perhaps of Victorian inspiration, and age for at least two days before use.

Scheherazade

When capricious Carnation flirts with stately Sandalwood, patrician Patchouli, beguiling Bergamot and seditious Cedarwood, their joint offspring is a witty and seductive fragrance as bewitching as Scheherazade herself. Combine in the mixing bottle one part (6 drops) of oil of Cedarwood, two parts Patchouli, three parts each of Sandalwood and Carnation and five parts of

Bergamot. Top up with diluent. By the time it took Scheherazade to twice captivate her husband with her stories, her eponymous fragrance will have blended to perfumed perfection.

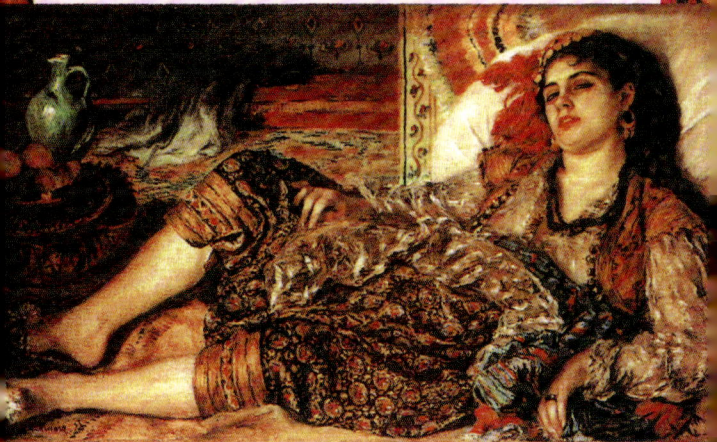

Postscript Pity poor Montaigne. For the sixteenth-century French essayist to have penned the words:

> *When smells a woman purely well?*
> *When she of nothing else does smell.*

he must never have been privy to his or any other lady's scented boudoir. *Le Pauvre!*

FRAGRANT WATERS

To succumb to the gentle, **Teasing Touch** of a skilled aromatherapist's **Firm Fingers** is the very **Pinnacle** of **Pleasure,** but before looking at the Whys and Wherefores of Massage, let us first reveal a few other means by which essential oils may be enjoyed.

The Aromatic Bath

Bathing in warm, scented waters and Breathing Deep the aroma of a blend of essential oils is one of the most blissful of aromatherapeutic benefits, for these oils can **Relax** or **Invigorate, Enhance** a Feeling of Wellbeing or Induce a Sense of Self-Esteem.

Warm compresses are made by floating a small towel or lint on sufficient hot water to which an Appropriate Oil has been added. Remove the material when it is saturated, wring out surplus water, and place the warm, scented cloth over the afflicted area. When the compress has cooled to Body Temperature, remove it and repeat the process until the pain has dissolved.

Cold compresses are made in an **Identical Fashion** using ice-cold rather than hand-hot water. The compress is effective until it has Heated to Body Temperature.

Once the bath has been struck, add up to six drops of either a favourite single oil or a **Bountiful Blend**, then disperse the oils through the steaming waters by swirling them with the hand. To add the oil while the taps are running causes much of the goodness to evaporate before you slip into the caressing water.

A Scented Shower

Once Basic Ablutions are completed, tarry awhile under the invigorating cascade and sprinkle up to three drops of a desired oil onto a thoroughly wet sponge or flannel and rub it all over your body. Do not be tempted to apply the oil directly to the skin. Breathe deeply for a few minutes and step from the shower a new person.

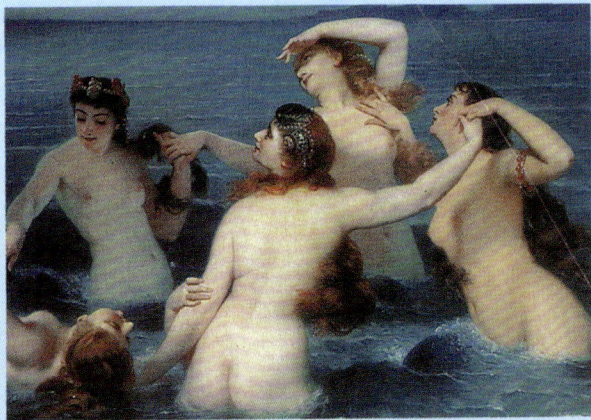

Inhalation

Grandmama was probably unaware that she was prac-
tising aromatherapy when she held the heads of the
young afflicted by colds over a bowl of Steaming Water to which she had added a magical mixture of oils,
whose components were a Treasured Family Secret.

Tissue inhalation

A drop or two of any suitable essential oil dabbed onto
a handkerchief or paper tissue can have a **Calming Effect** during crises that occur when travelling, perhaps
when one's postillion has been struck by lightning.

Footbaths

Steeping the feet (or hands) in a bowl of hand-hot water
to which four to six drops of an appropriate oil have
been added wards off chills and brings **Welcome Relief** to rheumatism, pain caused by arthritis, chilblains
and athlete's foot.

Compresses

Sooth muscular pains, sprains and bruises with an Ar-
omatically treated Compress; Cold for sprains, bruises, swellings, inflammations and headaches, Warm for
muscular pain, toothache, boils and abscesses. Warm
compresses can also be advocated for those of the **Fair
Sex** afflicted with menstrual cramp and cystitis.

NEROLI

How appropriate that this noble oil extracted from the bitter orange tree is named after a woman of noble birth - the Princess Anne Marie de la Tremoille de Neroli: how inappropriate that at one time in its history it was sported by women of ill virtue in Madrid to enable the men who sought their favours to identify them.

Neroli is an Anti-depressant of Some Significance: three drops mixed into two teaspoonsfuls of almond oil and rubbed clockwise onto the solar plexus, nape of the neck and temples, and then breathed in deeply for ten minutes banishes depression in Miraculous Fashion. Those who find sleep Elusive should seek Relief by adding a few drops of neroli oil to a warm bath.

Neroli oil is suitable for most skin types, but those with skins of Some Sensitivity should take care to use it only in the lowest concentration - one drop to three teaspoons of carrier oil is of sufficient strength. Numbered among Neroli's admirers was Marie Antoinette, the much-maligned queen of Louis XVI, who is reputed to have asked for her favourite oil on the eve of her fatal appointment with Madame Guillotine.

PATCHOULI

The oil obtained by distilling the Dried Leaves and Shoots of this highly odoriferous plant - a native to Malaysia - is one of the few that improves with age; a twenty-year-old essence being as Highly Prized to its owner as a Claret of similar vintage to an Oenophile.

It was once usual for Indian shawls imported into the British Isles to be scented with Patchouli; so appealing was this practice to aristocratic noses that weavers in the fair town of Paisley had to similarly scent their shawls in order to sell them.

Used sparingly in a pot pourri, it fills a room with its unmistakable bouquet, and those who wish their correspondence to linger fragrantly in the minds of its recipients will find that a few drops added to a bottle of Ink of a Proprietary Nature not only lends its fragrance to their letters, but also encourages the ink to dry.

Aromatherapists use patchouli to allay anxiety and depression, to counter oily skins and to encourage the growth of healthy, beautifully conditioned hair. Those plagued with unsightly acne should apply an admixture of grapeseed oil, wheatgerm oil and patchouli to the freshly-washed affected area morning and evening.

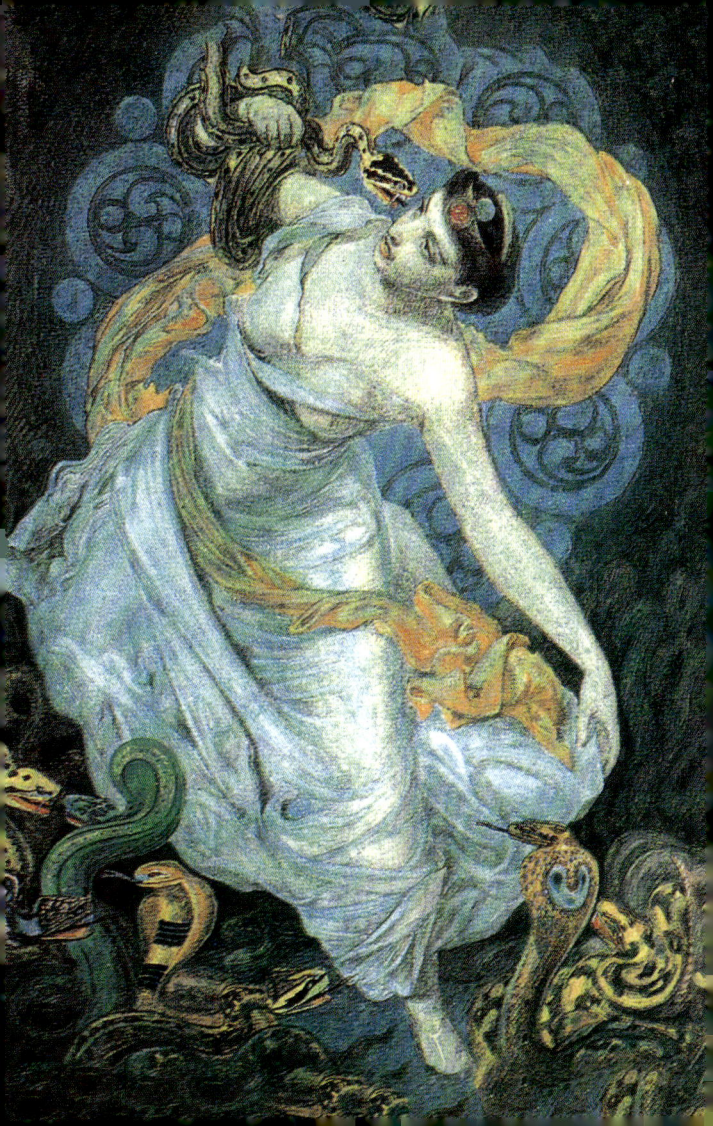

SCENTED SURROUNDINGS

Many and various are the **Fragrances** and **Moods** you can create in banishing stale air from the nooks and crannies of your house. Many and various are the means at your disposal in so doing, but one of the simplest and most effective of all is to fill a mist-spray bottle with distilled water and add some essential oils, to spray the air with a rich sprinkling of the beauty.

To fill a room with Forest Fragrance, pour four fluid ounces of distilled water into the bottle and add fifty drops of spruce, twenty-five drops each of lavender and eucalyptus and twenty of cedarwood. You will almost hear the crunch of pine needles beneath your feet as you stroll from desk to decanter.

For a Spicier Atmosphere, spray a mixture of the same amount of water into which you have rained ten drops of lime, fifteen of clove, twenty each of ginger, cinnamon and anise, and thirty-five of caraway. To close your eyes and breathe in deeply is to be carried away to a Zanzibar spice market where a clamour of aromas compete for your attention.

Enjoy an Imaginary Stroll round a Favourite Flower Garden awash with colourful, heavily scented blooms by misting the room with ten drops of jasmine, fifteen of cinnamon, twenty of clove, twenty five of rose and fifty of orange, all shaken into four fluid ounces (110ml) of distilled water.

And those who find that a Lemony Tang adds zest to their lives need do no more than mix ten drops each of patchouli and orange, fifty of grapefruit and the same amount of lime, again with four fluid ounces of distilled water and mist the room accordingly.

A Refreshing Minty Atmosphere can be achieved by spraying an admixture of four fluid ounces of distilled water with ten drops each of lime, peppermint and benzoin, twenty of rosemary, thirty of lavender and forty of spearmint. Filling the lungs with air freshened with this intoxicating aroma clears the head gloriously and encourages you to face anything the world may care to throw at you.

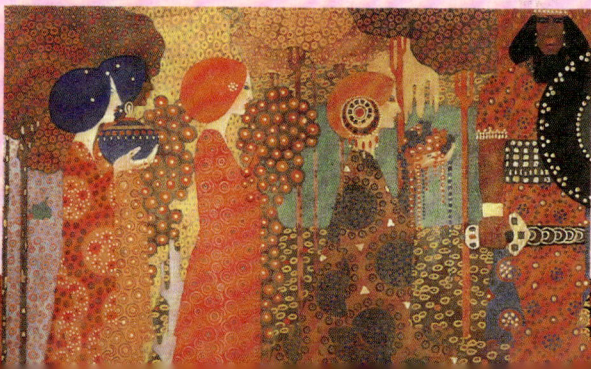

ROSEMARY

Culpeper held that rosemary '*quickens a weak memory and the senses*', and indeed is one of the three **Celaphic Herbs,** basil and peppermint being the other two, credited with the capacity to stimulate the brain thus encouraging clarity of thought and freshness of memory.

Rosemary was sacred to the **Greeks** and **Romans,** both civilisations believing it symbolized love and death and for centuries has been used in **Marriage Ceremonies** and **Funerary Rites.**

The warm camphorous smell and the Remarkable Potency of the oil extracted from the hardy evergreen shrub make it a favourite in the Aromatherapy Larder. Indeed it is of such potency that it must not be used in any concentration, no matter how weak, during the first trimester of pregnancy.

Those who are not with child may safely look to rosemary to treat arthritis, bronchitis, burns, colds and influenza. It can help reduce overhigh cholesterol levels and increase low blood pressure. Those who are oft laid low with a pounding migraine, could well look to rosemary for relief. But it is probably in matters concerning the hair and scalp that rosemary oil is put to best use.

And now, having sung its praises, it must be pointed out that if used in too high a concentration, or over a long period of time, rosemary may adversely affect those subject to *petit* or *grand mal*.

It is an oil of sociable nature and blends well with basil, cedarwood, coriander, frankincense, juniper, lavender and peppermint, and is especially fond of the citrus oils.

To Poor Tragic Ophelia, Rosemary was for remembrance. To aromatherapists the world over it is a boon and blessing.

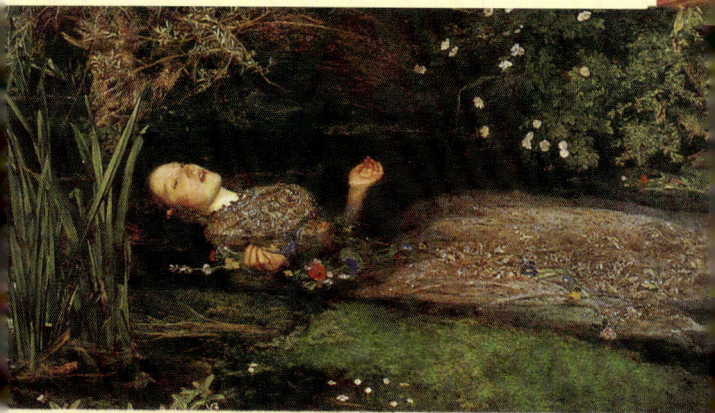

FLICKERING FRAGRANCES

A room lit with candles rests the eye and soothes the mind. **Candlelight** is flattering especially for those who having reached a Certain Age are no longer in the first flush of youth. Add to the atmosphere by dripping several drops of an aromatic oil onto the wax before lighting the candle: never let the oil come into contact with the wick for some oils are of a highly inflammable nature.

For a citrus scent, use grapefruit, lemon, lemongrass, lime, melissa, neroli or orange.

If you prefer a floral aroma try benzoin, jasmine, rose, tolu balsam or ylang-ylang.

For an invigorating forest perfume use eucalyptus, myrtle, pine, rosemary or spruce.

Peppermint and spearmint fill the room with a delightful minty fragrance, and allspice, caraway, clove and sage add spice to the atmosphere.

Celebrate **Easter** with a joyful mix of equal quantities of coriander, geranium and ylang ylang, and hail **Midsummer** with a happy marriage of bergamot and juniper, or angelica and lemon, all in equal quantities. At **Harvest Time** bring Nature's bounty into your house by burning candles aglow with bergamot, grapefruit and orange in equal quantities with a lesser amount of frankincese. Heighten the mystery of **Hallowe'en** with candles bursting with cedarwood, clary sage and vetiver, or clary sage and patchouli with a dash of vetiver. The Aged Crones who haunt the skies on the eve of All Saints' Day could produce no better as they mount their broomsticks ready to take flight into the night.

At **Christmas** use a mixture of equal quantities of cedarwood, frankincense and myrrh (or if this is too much for your taste, lighten the scent by adding a few drops of bergamot, mandarin or orange). And what could be more appropriate than to use candles of a golden hue to celebrate the Epiphany.

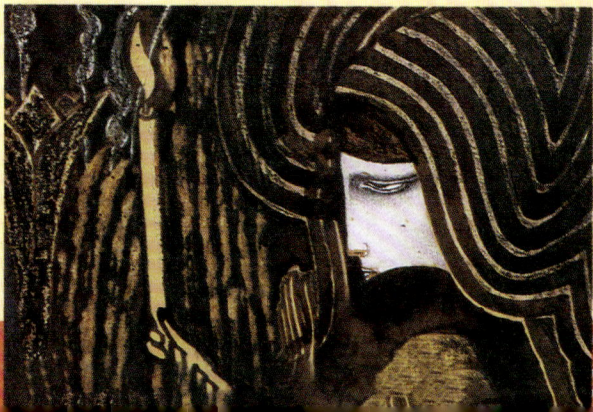

ROSE OTTO

Was the rose created from a Drop of Sweat that fell from Mohammed's brow? Or did appreciative Bacchus cause a thorny bush to be covered with red flowers when the object of his lust caught herself on its thorns and revealed even more of her sumptuous beauty.

According to Indian legend, the Princess Nour-Djiban was so in love with her Mogul groom that she ordered the canals in her garden to be filled with rosewater in which the adoring couple rowed in fragrant bliss until they noticed a green oil floating on the surface. The heat of the sun had fused the rosewater's fragrant molecules: Glorious essential Rose Otto oil had been created. A Delightful Tale, but told at least eight centuries after the Greek physician Galen had recommended the addition of rose essential oil to a cold cream of his creation.

The extravagantly expensive oil marries happily with bergamot, chamomile, cedarwood, clary sage, frankincense, patchouli, sandalwood, vetiver and ylang-ylang and is so wondrously concentrated that only the tiniest drop should be used if it is not to dominate the others into fragrant submission.

It is not just the oil that has come to be held in such High Esteem. Rosewater, too, is a trusted friend. It is extremely effective for eye complaints, especially Irritating Conjunctivitis and is a cooling, refreshing and charmingly scented skin toner.

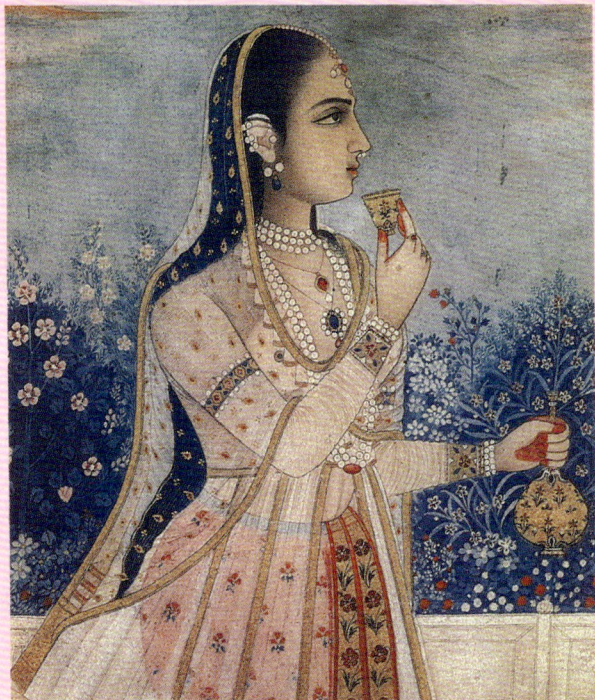

Aromatherapy in the Workplace

The modern workplace, be it Bureau, Emporium or Factory, is a place of stress and friction. The pressure to succeed in the Hothouse Atmosphere where very survival is often a challenge is intense. Aromatherapy can help us all to take these stresses in our stride and to rise above them on a Delicately Scented Cloud.

Those fortunate enough to have their **Own Space** in which to work can select the oils that suit them best. Those who work alongside others should consider the Feelings of their Colleagues and gain their approval before introducing them to the delights of Mood-enhancing Aromas. It may take several attempts to find a fragrance that is acceptable to the olfactory organs of all, but it is well worth the time this may take.

The ways in which the perfumes may be diffused are several: a simple bowl of Pot-pourri on which a few drops of a favourite oil have been sprinkled may be appropriate; a small bowl of a suitable mixture of oils rested atop a heating source, will sweeten the air and banish Dame Stress; similarly a **light bulb ring**, a Hollowed-out Brass Contraption that rests on top of an electric light bulb, diffuses the aroma of the oil within when the bulb is hot.

The more Affluent may consider the purchase of a handsome, ornamental earthenware **Vaporizer**, or even a new-fangled **Electric Fragrancer.**

Which fragrances to use? Experience suggests that the most enhancing aromas for the Work Environment are those either of the Green Family which are redolent of Pine, Cypress and Juniper: or its sister Citrus with her tangy Lemon, Orange, Lime and Grapefruit fragrances.

To close the eyes for a second and breathe deeply of the aromatic air, is to leave the Hustle and Bustle of the workplace behind for a refreshing moment or two. A blend of either Cypress, Petitgrain and Bergamot, or one of Pine, Eucalyptus and Lemon will send the imagination on an invigorating stroll through Scented Groves: while Lavender, Rosemary and Grapefruit combine to create the crystal-clarity of the air in an Alpine Meadow.

Aromatherapy in the workplace can also help to maintain a healthy atmosphere, preventing the spread of bacteria. Oil of Eucalyptus and Tea Tree are exceedingly effective allies in the **fight** against the **coughs** and **sneezes** that plague us so during the Winter Months. If their aroma is not to the liking of all, they can be blended with Lemon or Lavender.

For those seeking mental stimulation, Peppermint, Rosemary and Basil encourage clear thinking, as do a mixture of Basil, Bergamot and Coriander, an amalgam of Juniper and Lemon and a marriage of Eucalyptus, Grapefruit and Bergamot.

The creation of such a Soothing Atmosphere will be Conducive of Great Productivity in all areas of Effort.

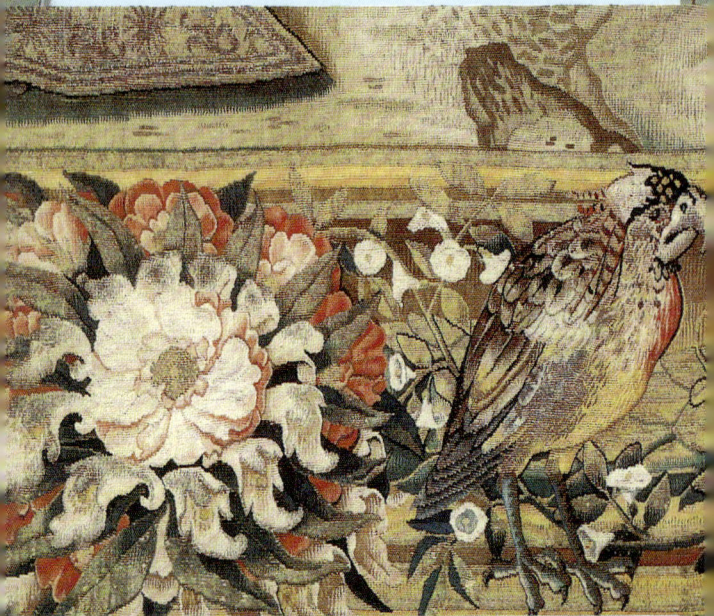

SANDALWOOD

No Oriental Perfume is complete without Sandalwood: no Aromatherapist's Larder is complete without a phial of the softly woody essential oil that lingers in the air as evocatively as a Lover's Unseen Glance.

Sandalwood is mentioned in Sanskrit and Chinese documents. **Ancient Egyptians** burned it to venerate their gods. Sandalwood paste was rubbed into the foreheads of **Hindu Priests** as a mark of their spiritual purity and practitioners of Indian holistic medicine have long used sandalwood in their lotions and potions.

The oil is now mainly extracted from sawdust and woodchippings from the woodmills of India. But, *alas*, the trees so processed take up to seventy years to grow to full maturity and their very popularity has led to large-scale destruction of the sandalwood plantations there.

To show our concern for Our Environment we should be sparing in our use of sandalwood oil – indeed many aromatherapists now refrain from using it, preferring instead to resort to a suitable substitute. That said, sheets kept in a linen fold carved from sandalwood have a sleep-inducing fragrance that approaches the divine.

BANISH TIRESOME BUGS!

A child of One's Acquaintance was heard to ask its Flustered Parent, 'Mummy, what are insects for?' Whereupon the Flustered Parent suggested that perhaps her offspring would be happier in the Nursery with Nanny.

The Almighty could no doubt account for insects in His Great Scheme of Things, but to those of us who are not privy to His Plan, insects remain a tiresome nuisance. Thankfully, several Essential Oils have valuable Repellent Properties and the Aromatherapist's Receipt Book has several remedies for the treatment of insect bites and stings.

Five drops of either geranium, chamomile or lavender oils added to a teaspoonful of aloe vera gel may be safely applied to the site of an insect bite every few hours.

Lavender is a worthy ally in skirmishes against the Insectavora. It is one of the few oils which may be safely applied neat to an insect bite and will cause any pain to vanish in seconds. A pot of lavender keeps flies and moths at bay. A scrap of paper impregnated with a mixture of citrus oil and lavender is a marvellous weapon against Mother Moth's Tenacious Teeth.

Geranium oil is another fragrant ally. Rubbing a tincture composed of four teaspoons of soya oil and sixteen drops of geranium oil over the body before Venturing Forth keeps most insects at bay.

Essential oils are also Sturdy Soldiers in the gardeners' infantry. Watering plants with a solution of five drops of lavender, ten drops of thyme in a sufficiency of water, agitated thoroughly to ensure that the oils are well dispersed, should keep most plants insect free. So, too, will five drops of clove and ten of sage oils mixed with an amplitude of water and Rained Regularly over the garden.

For plants already infested, stronger treatment is advocated. Misting a plant with a spray composed of fifty drops of lavender, forty of fennel and four fluid ounces of water, should rid the beastly blight.

HERE'S THE RUB

Having one's muscles massaged whilst inhaling the fragrance of the essential oils being rhythmically rubbed into the body is wondrous in the extreme. That these oils could pass directly through the skin was once a matter of Much Dispute but anyone who refuses to believe that just as the skin eliminates, it can absorb, need do no more than rub cut garlic cloves over the soles of feet: their scepticism is sure to dissolve when, within the space of a few hours the unmistakable smell of garlic will be lingering on their breath.

To pay homage to Mother Science, massage assists in the elimination of toxic wastes which relieves muscular pain by increasing nutrition to painful areas of the body. As body tensions are released, so fear, anxiety and other negative emotions dissolve into Sweet Nothingness, and by combining Madame Massage with the Sister Subtleties of essential oils, the fortunate person being massaged may be influenced on many different levels.

Avoid giving or receiving a massage under the harsh artificial, electric light. Intensify the atmosphere by illumining the Massage Parlour with candles, or drape the lamps with cloth of a Soothing Hue.

Before the massage your Aromamasseur (or indeed Aromasseuse) will decide on the oil or blend of oils to be used to make sure that they are diluted in a suitable base oil in the Proper Proportions. Concentrations of between half and one per cent should be used for facial massage or if using Basil, Chamomile, Fennel, Ginger, Lemon Grass or Melissa. In no circumstance should a concentration of more than three per cent be used.

It is not possible for us, given the Constraints of Space, to Effect an Introduction to Myriad Blends that can be prepared to relieve aches and pains, to calm, to Relax the muscles, to increase Physical Endurance and Banish Stress, to refresh and to Encourage Romance.

Mother Nature has endowed us with such a wealth of oils that there is sure to be an admixture that is just right for you, so by all means follow the advice offered by that master of the Lithesome Lyric, Cole Porter, who wrote in his musical extravaganza, *Nymph Errant* 'the apple at the top of the tree is never too high to achieve, So take an example from Eve, *Experiment . . .*'

Do so, Dear Reader, but do so with care.

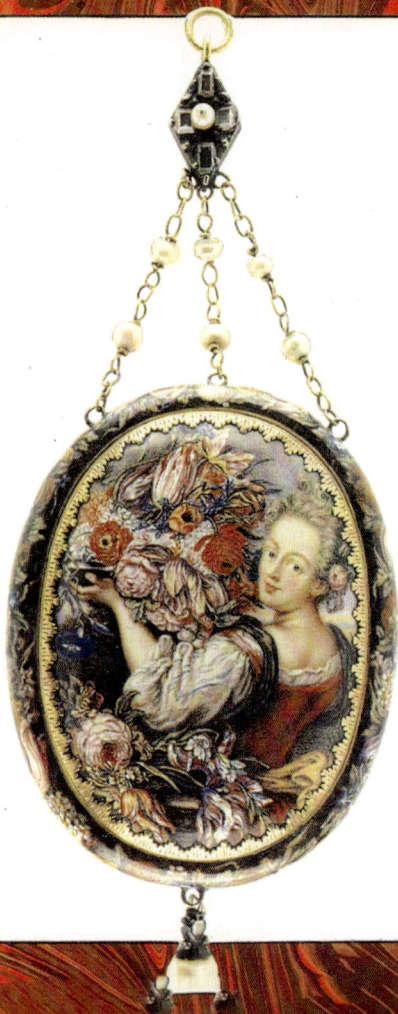